fleur de force

The Luxe Life

First published in 2016 by
HEADLINE PUBLISHING GROUP

1

Designed by Siobhan Hooper
All Photography by Laurie Fletcher and Fleur De Force except as follows:
Shutterstock.com: p. 3 © davorna, p. 103 © All About Space, p. 105 © Chaikom, p. 113 © Anna
    Ismagilova, p. 234 © Anna Ok, p. 237 © NY Studio, p. 245 © Anna-Mari West, p. 247 (all)
    © kikovic, p. 249 © ouh_desire
p. 42 © Robert Przybysz/Alamy
p. 129 © Bob Barkany/Getty Images
p. 216 © John Alexander Photography – www.jeaphotography.co.uk
Illustrations by Yoco Nagamiya
Hair Styling by Gareth Smith
Clothes Styling by Emily Giffard-Taylor
Food Styling by Warren 'Ollie' Hoile
Cakes on p. 189, 191, 192 and 194 baked by Emily Laramy

Hardback ISBN 978 1 4722 3206 9

Printed and bound in Italy by Rotolito Lombarda S.p.A.

Headline's policy is to use papers that are natural, renewable and recyclable products and made from wood grown in well-managed forests and other controlled sources. The logging and manufacturing processes are expected to conform to the environmental regulations of the country of origin.

HEADLINE PUBLISHING GROUP
An Hachette UK Company
Carmelite House
50 Victoria Embankment
London EC4Y 0DZ

www.headline.co.uk

www.hachette.co.uk

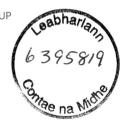

For my mum, the best host, all-round inspiration
and best friend I've ever had.
Thanks for teaching me how to have fun.

Contents

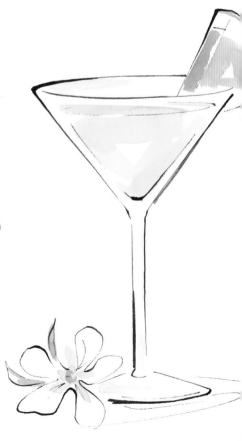

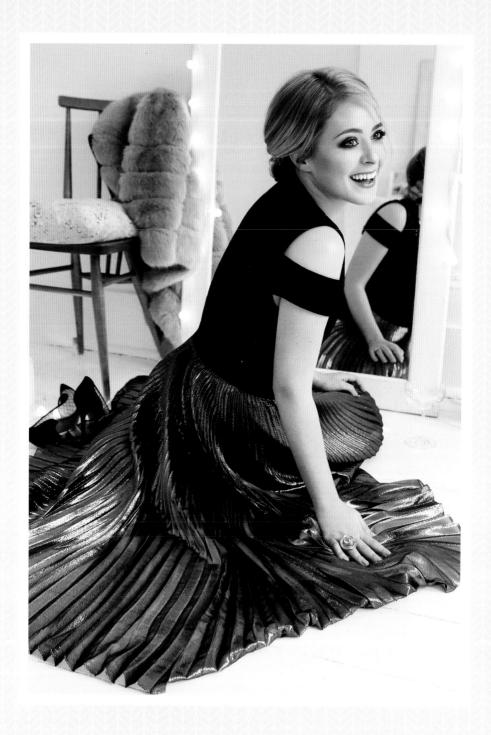

Introduction

Some of my earliest memories involve my mum hosting huge dinner parties at home. I used to love helping her prepare the food, lay the table and helping her choose outfits and get ready (and even more so snacking on the delicious leftovers the day after!) I think, through her, my life has always involved entertaining. and it's something that comes naturally to me, but that I also adore. Now I'm an adult and have my own home, I still love hosting and entertaining and everything that comes with it.

I've also always been obsessed with gift giving, choosing or making personalised gifts and wrapping them beautifully (from a young age I used to insist on wrapping all of my mum, grandma and brother's Christmas gifts in the run up to Christmas).

For my second book, I wanted to marry this passion for hosting, occasions and formalities with the beauty and fashion tips for wowing at special occasions I've learnt during the past six-and-a-half years I've been making beauty videos on YouTube. My debut book *The Glam Guide* was all about the basics for a glam life, from beauty and fashion to healthy living and positive thinking. *The Luxe Life* is its more sophisticated, older sister and in it I hope to share with you all my top tips and secrets for making the most of every occasion to dress up, host a party or buy the perfect present. You don't have to be rolling in cash to live a 'luxe' life, it's all about going that extra mile to make every occasion extra special.

Black-Tie Beauty

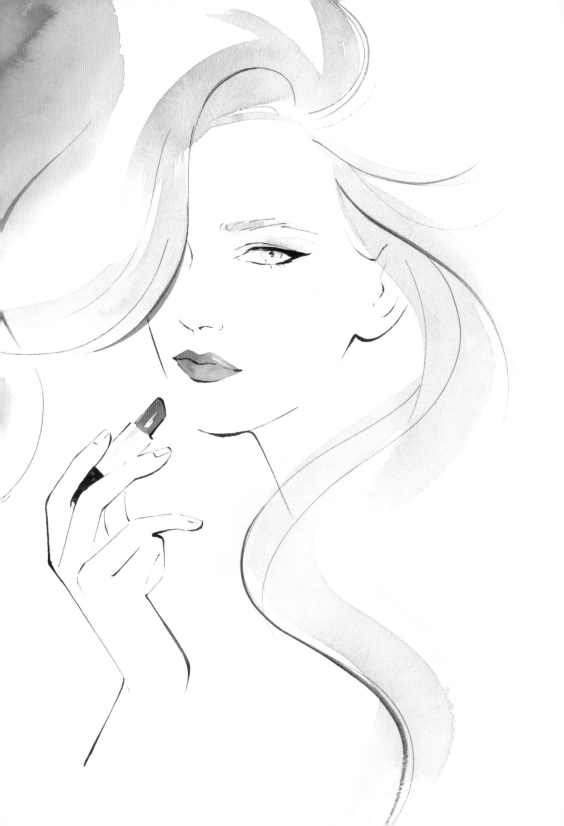

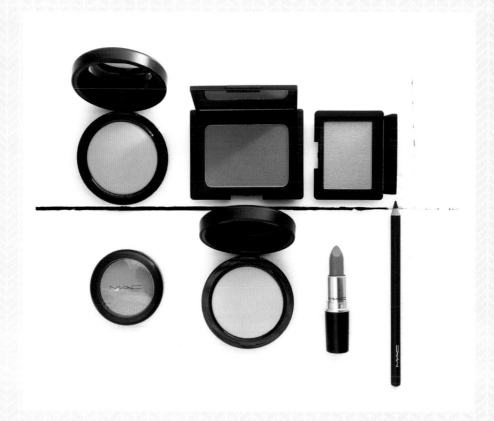

How to Make Your Makeup Last

One of the questions I get asked most frequently is how to make your makeup last all day. Whether it's by a bride ahead of her wedding day, a friend before a night out or one of my viewers who works long hours and doesn't want to worry about touching-up her makeup every few hours. Whatever your reason for wanting to know, the following tips and tricks can help to make your life a whole lot less high-maintenance when it comes to makeup.

Prep

Prepping your skin before makeup application is one of the best ways to ensure your makeup lasts as long as possible, and also to help make it look its very best. Make sure your skin is well moisturised before applying any primer or foundation, and also ensure that any product is fully absorbed into the skin. However, try to avoid overloading your skin with product, especially around the eye area, as it will prevent your makeup from applying perfectly.

Prime

While the world of primers, bases and makeup-setting sprays can seem confusing, investing in the right ones can help make your life much easier and your makeup last much longer. These products have exploded in popularity over the past few years and there are now so many to choose from, making it hard to know which ones actually work without wasting your money testing them all out. When it comes to foundation primers, my favourites are from Laura Mercier (who also make a great oil-free option for those with oily skin), Lancôme and Soap & Glory. For eye primers, it doesn't get much better than Urban Decay's cult Primer Potion, which now comes in a few different shades as well as the original nude one. If you want to skip a step and use a cream eye shadow as a base, this works really well if you have the right shadow. My personal favourites are the Laura Mercier Caviar Stick Eye Colour. As for makeup-setting sprays, despite being a totally different concept to a powder, they really do work and are a great option for those with dry skin. They are also great to have in your bag to use throughout the day to help keep your makeup looking fresh, and help avoid any makeup build-up from using powder, which can make your foundation look cakey. When it comes to powder, when used sparingly it's your best bet when it comes to keeping shine at bay on oily skins. Using powder to set your makeup is essential for longevity, but you may want to invest in some blotting sheets before powdering throughout the day, as this will absorb any excess oil (which may result in the kind of shine you don't want) and also help your makeup to last longer.

Layer

Apply your makeup in thin layers, allowing any liquid products to dry fully before applying the next layer, building up the colour as you go. This technique takes longer but ensures longevity and works equally well with foundation, eye shadow and blush.

Set

When layering, make sure you think about textures when determining the order in which you apply your products. Cream and liquid products should always be applied before powder products for the smoothest application and best finish. Set any cream products you use with powder to make them last as long as possible. This applies for all colour products: if you subtly layer cream blush, gel eyeliner or cream eye shadow underneath their powder counterparts, it will not only help them last longer but will also help intensify the colours too.

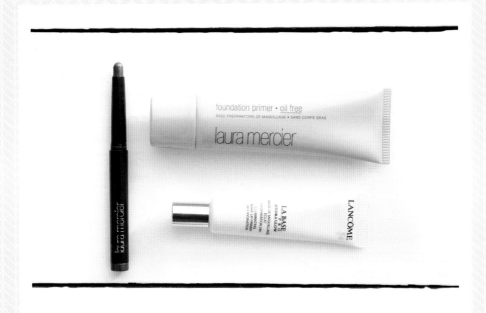

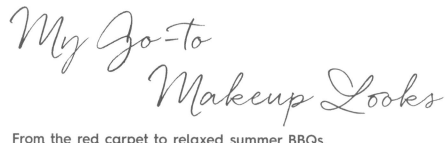

My Go-to Makeup Looks

**From the red carpet to relaxed summer BBQs,
these five looks have me covered for every occasion**

When I want to look my best for a special occasion, I have five go-to looks
I tend to gravitate towards. Remember there are no rights and wrongs when
it comes to makeup: it's all about working out what works best for you. These
are my personal favourites and keep me covered for all eventualities.

CLASSIC VINTAGE GLAMOUR

My first choice if I'm wearing an LBD, especially in the winter, although this
look works year-round.

* Contoured matte eye shadow
* Winged liquid liner
* Flawless skin
* Subtle blush
* Matte red lipstick

Additional extra

Natural-looking false lashes make an
elegant addition to this look. You don't
want to go for anything too dramatic,
as the winged liner and red lip is
already making quite a statement. I
usually go for the Simply Fleur design
from my range with Eylure.

Go-to products

* **Too Faced Born This Way foundation.** This gives a full coverage, with a glowing, flawless finish. I always lightly powder this foundation to set it, as it is quite a moveable formula.
* **Stila Stay All Day liquid eyeliner.** This is the longest-lasting eyeliner I've ever used. It has a glossy finish so is best used for more statement, glamorous looks. The felt-tip nib makes it easy to create the perfect winged look too.
* **Urban Decay's Naked 2 Basics Palette.** This is my failsafe when it comes to natural matte eye shadows. I like the second version better than the first as the shades are more neutral and cool-toned rather than warm. You can also use it for filling in your brows.
* **MAC's RiRi Woo lipstick.** The ultimate matte finish red. This is a universally flattering shade and the staying power is incredible.

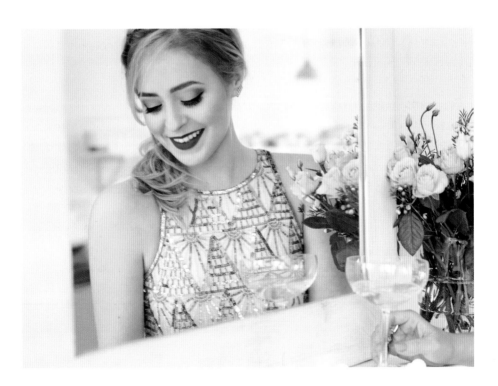

DAYTIME GLAMOUR

A pared-down version of the previous look, this is my go-to for daytime parties or events. It looks polished and glamorous, but still fresh and natural. This is without a doubt my most-worn look of them all, as well as being the quickest and easiest if you're short on time.

* Light and fresh-looking base makeup
* Subtle blush and slight contouring of the cheeks with luminous highlights
* Natural pink-mauve lipstick
* Little-flick winged eyeliner
* Messy voluminous lashes

Go-to products

* **Chanel Vitalumière Aqua foundation.** Possibly my all-time favourite foundation, this is ultra-light and cooling on the skin. The coverage is buildable so you can choose the level you want or need.
* **Hourglass Ambient Lighting blushes and powders.** Uniquely subtle and beautiful, these blushes are natural yet leave a glowing effect on the skin, and the powders are stunning when used to highlight the high points of the face. They are expensive, but last a long time so are well worth the investment if you're looking for the best-quality powders around.

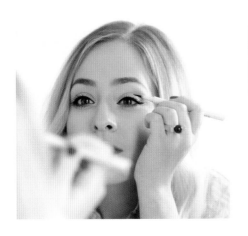

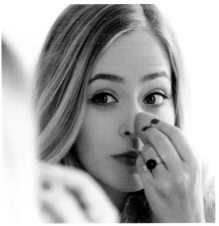

★ **Fleur De Force Beauty Written in the Stars lip gloss.** This product from my own line is the perfect daytime shade to look polished yet natural.

★ **Topshop Magic Liner.** A great option for daytime liquid liner. It has impressive staying power, a nice demi-matte finish and easy application.

★ **Max Factor Masterpiece mascara.** One of my favourite options for naturally voluminous lashes with just the right level of definition.

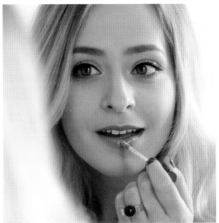

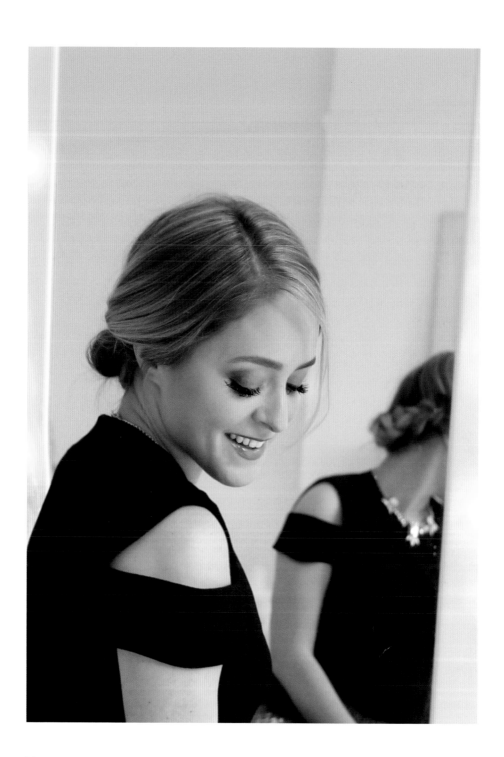

CLASSIC SMOKY EYE

A lot of people's favourite evening look. I wanted to include it here as it's a very versatile look, and everyone has their own take on it and different tweaks and techniques. I tend to wear a smoky eye on summer evenings but it's a great look to master as you can tweak it to create so many different variations very easily.

* Flawless semi-matte skin
* Natural-toned blush with subtle contouring
* Natural or nude glossy lips
* Matte smoky eye blended with pale or white matte shades on the inner corner of the eye and brow bone
* Black kohl pencil liner on the waterline of the eye
* Lashings of black mascara

Additional extra

I don't like using full-on false lashes with smoky eyes as it can easily look too much, but I love using three-quarter-length lashes to accentuate the shape of the eyes and add volume and a pretty flutter. My favourites for this are my Fleur Loves lashes. For particularly glittering events, I also like to introduce different shimmery colour to the centre of the eyelid; loose glitter pigments or highly pigmented pressed powders are great for this. Urban Decay make my favourites.

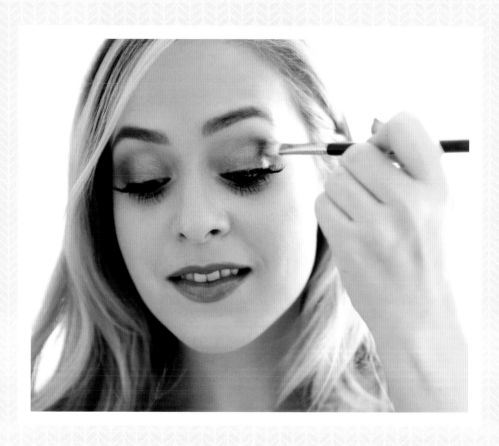

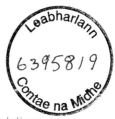

Go-to products

* **Bourjois Air Mat foundation.** One of the best matte-finish foundations on the high street, this is matte but doesn't look flat and is great quality for the price too.

* **MAC's Blush Baby.** When you're going bold on your eyes, you want to keep it simple for the rest of the look. This shade is great as it's a natural-toned flush and doesn't have any shimmer so looks as natural as possible, but still adds definition.

* **Maybelline Master Sculpt Duo.** This contouring duo is great for those new to contouring. Apply the darker colour in the hollows of your cheeks, at your temples, down the side of your nose, underneath your jawline and down each side of your neck to make your bone structure appear sharper and your face slimmer (if you want to know more about contouring and my top tips and tricks, there a whole chapter on it in my previous book, *The Glam Guide*).

* **MAC's Patisserie lipstick.** I don't like pale nude lips; I prefer to keep them looking natural, yet perfected. MAC's Patisserie is a little darker and has a lustre finish, so it has a light gloss to it that works really well with a smoky eye.

* **Urban Decay's Naked palettes.** The Naked palettes are my favourites for creating smoky eye looks as they all have a great black shade, a selection of paler matte and shimmery tones, and the formulas are second to none. Choose one based on your skin tone and preferences (Naked 1 is warm or brown-based, 2 is cool or grey-based and 3 is pink-based).

* **Rimmel's Scandaleyes eyeliner pencil.** This eyeliner is a makeup bag staple for me. It's extremely black and blendable, but stays put after it has dried and is really long-lasting. Don't waste your money buying expensive eyeliners: the best high-street equivalents are often the same or better quality.

* **YSL's Effet Faux Cils Shocking mascara.** This is without a doubt my favourite mascara when it comes to building up a ridiculous level of volume.

RELAXED SMOKY LOOK

The perfect alternative for those who don't like the heavy look of a full-on smoky eye, or if you want to rock a smoky eye in the daytime, this look is a lighter alternative to the full-on smoky eye and works really well for all-day wear and for a more casual look. It's also easier to pair with a bold lipstick without looking 'too much'.

* Natural, fresh-looking base makeup
* A glowing peach-toned blusher with a slight shimmer
* Neutral-toned brown eye shadow as a base, blended with a light matte shade on the inner corner and brow bone
* A thick line of brown eye pencil or crème eye shadow along the upper and lower lash line, blended out using a small pencil brush to create a subtle smoky look that is most concentrated along the lashes (rather than the outer corner of the eye as with the full-on smoky look)
* Your favourite lipstick. This look is quite versatile, so it goes with lots of different lip shades. My personal favourite is a natural mauve, glossy look

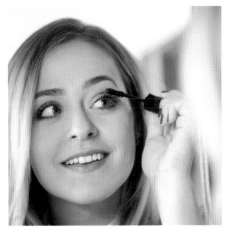

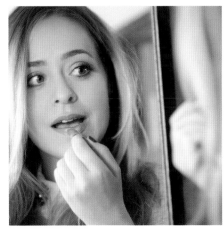

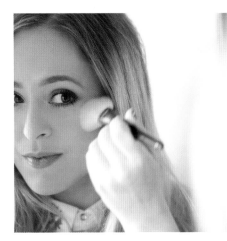

Go-to products

★ **Bourjois' 123 Perfect CC cream.**
This is my favourite base for this
look as it gives a good level
of coverage while still looking
really natural on the skin. It's got
a moisturising formula so stays
looking fresh throughout the day.

★ **NARS Orgasm powder blush.** This
is the best peach-toned blusher I
own. It looks natural and glowing,
but has a subtle shimmer to it that
looks really glam.

★ **Urban Decay's Naked 1 palette.**
The Naked 1 is the perfect palette
for this kind of look, but I do also
love using the Laura Mercier Caviar
Stick Eye Colour for blending along
the lash line.

SUMMER BRONZE

There's nothing better than going full-on bronzed when you've got a bit of a tan in the summertime. It looks glamorous yet natural, and is a great way to accentuate your features.

* A glowing, dewy base makeup. Tinted moisturisers work really well for this
* A shimmery bronzer placed carefully along the high points of the face (think of applying it in a 'E3' motion over your forehead, cheekbones and jaw line). Having a slight shimmer to the bronzer will mean you'll get that tanned effect as well as adding a highlight when the high points of your face catch the light
* A cream eye shadow in a warm brown or bronze shade. I usually just use one colour for this kind of look
* A messy, blended out dark brown eyeliner
* Lots of mascara
* Your favourite natural/nude lipstick

Go-to products

* **Laura Mercier's tinted moisturiser** is my favourite in the summertime. They also make an oil-free version, and an illuminating one with a bit of shimmer in it that can look really beautiful with a tan.
* I'm loving the **Hourglass Ambient Lighting bronzer** at the moment. It's the perfect choice for a look like this as it has shimmer to it but it's not 'too much'.
* **Bobbi Brown** makes some of the best cream eye shadows on the market. Her long-wear cream formulas are available in both pots and pencils and they are both equally as lovely.
* **MAC's Coffee eyeliner** is my favourite liner for this look as it's really dark. Some browns don't show up very well, this one really adds definition without being black.
* One of my favourite multi-use products that lends itself perfectly to this kind of look is **NARS' The Multiple in Laguna**. It's great because you can use it as a bronzer, eye shadow and even a lip tint.

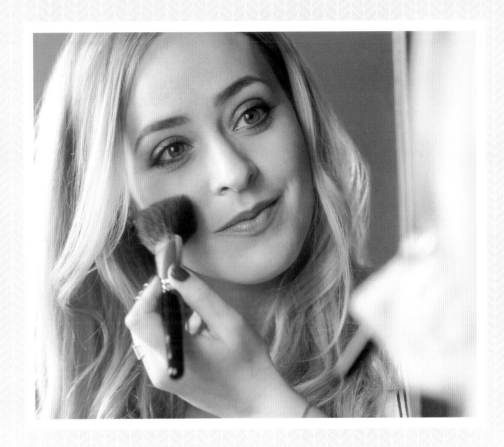

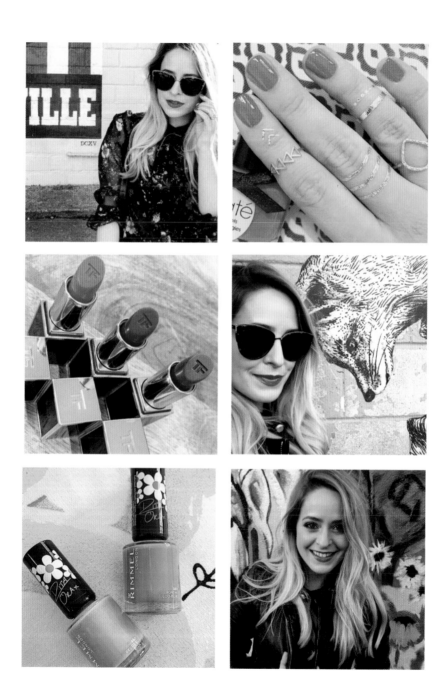

How to Wear Colour (and Own It!)

So many of my friends and family shy away from brightly coloured makeup – even red lipstick. As an avid bright lip fan, this really surprises me, but when I think back to the first time I ever wore a red lipstick, I do remember feeling overly self-conscious. So how do you learn to be comfortable with colour? Here are my top tips for wearing colour, and owning it.

Introduce it gradually

If you're not used to wearing bold colours, introduce them gradually into your makeup arsenal. Try out a mid-toned pink first, then get brighter as your confidence grows, or try wearing it around the house to get used to it, and see how it wears over time, so you know when it might need touching up throughout the day when you do wear it out.

Stick to one colour at a time!

It's really tricky to pull off two bold colours at the same time, especially if they are in different areas, e.g. on the eyes and lips. So if you're experimenting with bold makeup, stick to just one colour at a time, keeping the rest of your makeup neutral.

Pick the right shade

Picking the right shade of colour to wear is so important, and links to your skin tone. There's a whole chapter on colours to suit your skin tone in my first book, so I'd recommend checking that out if you're unsure. But once you've established what suits you, stick to it.

Try accents of colour

Bright makeup can sometimes look a little childish if not worn well. A great tip to make it look more sophisticated is to stick to accent colours. One of my favourite looks for the eyes is to go for a bold eyeliner instead of a full eye shadow look. It's still visually striking, but in a much more subtle, stylish way.

Pair it with simple, chic clothing

Even the most perfectly applied, beautiful red lip can look garish if you pair it with the wrong outfit. Pair your bolder makeup choices with simple designs in classic colours that don't fight with the makeup, both in terms of colour and tone.

Don't forget to touch up!

Don't forget that brighter makeup often needs retouching a little more often throughout the day than more neutral choices. Especially when it comes to bold lips, it's worth having a little compact mirror on hand for on-the-go check-ups and post-meal touch-ups are a must. It will vary from product to product, and as you use them you'll get to know how frequently your favourite products need refreshing throughout the day.

Be confident

The number one most important advice for wearing bright makeup is to be confident about it. If you make the decision to walk out the door wearing red lipstick, or blue eyeliner, be confident in your decision and you'll easily pull it off.

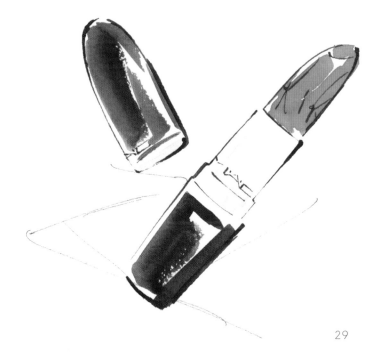

Day to Night
Essentials

We've all been there (probably more than a few times!): you've got five minutes in the back of a cab or the office bathroom to update your look from drab end-of-the-day makeup to polished and sophisticated, ready for a special event. Instead of slapping on the standard red lipstick, try the following ideas to instantly update your look, leaving you looking flawless and polished.

REFRESH YOUR BASE

Instead of simply layering on more concealer or powder over the top of my existing foundation, I like to apply a fresh layer of foundation if I can. I remove my existing base (avoiding the eyes) using micellar water or a face wipe, then apply an easy-to-blend foundation to refresh my base before applying any more makeup. This avoids any thick or cakey effect you might get from layering-up products.

My recommendation

Estée Lauder Double Wear Makeup to Go. This push-up compact version of Lauder's cult classic full-coverage foundation is a great handbag staple for updating your look as it's really versatile. It's full coverage, yet buildable, so you can layer it up to achieve a totally flawless look in the evening. You can also use it in place of concealer if you prefer a less full-coverage finish.

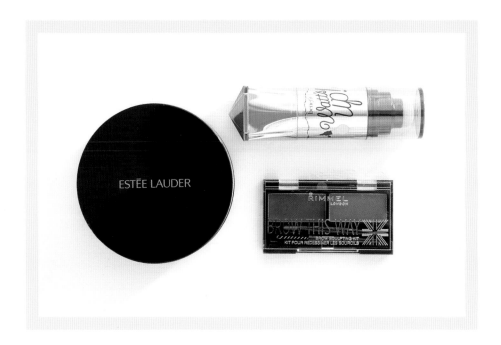

GIVE YOURSELF A GLOW

A perfectly placed highlighter in a subtle shade can instantly transform your makeup from tired to glamorous and glowing. Creams work really well for day-to-night looks as they are portable, multi-use and look fresh and light on the skin. I apply highlighter to the high points of my cheekbones, on my cupid's bow, brow bones and a tiny bit down the bridge of my nose. I also love using highlighters on my eyes if I'm in a hurry – they can work wonders used on the inner corners of the eyes to brighten them, or all over the eyelid for a subtle shimmer.

My recommendation

Benefit's Watt's Up! highlighter. This is a great product for day-to-night updates as it's packaged in a compact stick and has a little smudger on the end if you don't want to use your fingers to apply it on the go. It's a beautiful champagne colour that can look really subtle and natural, but it's also buildable for a more striking highlighted look in the evening.

DON'T FORGET
YOUR BROWS

Well-groomed brows can easily make any makeup look instantly more polished. One minute spent on your brows can help to pull your whole look together, so don't skip them if you're in a hurry!

My recommendation

Estee Lauder's Double Wear Brow Lift Duo. Perfect for doing your brows on the go, this double-ended pencil has both a darker shade for filling in your brows and a lighter shade for highlighting your brow bone and defining the shape of your brows. Using a lighter colour to define your brows makes them look extra polished in next to no time, so it's perfect for getting a flawless look in a few minutes. It's also super-slim and compact so great for your handbag too. If you are looking for a great one-stop shop product for your brows, try Rimmel's Brow This Way tinted brow gel. It give your brows volume and colour and sets them in place all at the same time – a perfect option if you're short on time.

REMEMBER, THE
STATEMENT LIP IS
OPTIONAL

The typical day-to-night look usually involves slapping on a statement lip, but you're better off focusing on what suits you and applying it well rather than simply grabbing a red lipstick (it's likely you'll end up with it on your teeth if you're in a hurry anyway!). I prefer to stick to my favourite neutral shades. Layering-up a gloss over a lipstick also helps to add dimension and depth to the lips. If you want to go for bright, make sure it's a tried-and-tested formula you know is going to last (if you're short on time, you don't want to be worrying about it transferring everywhere!).

My recommendations

I love MAC's Patisserie layered underneath Written in the Stars from my makeup line. For red you can't go wrong with MAC's RiRi Woo. It's a universally flattering red with an ultra-matte finish. Once it's on, it isn't budging.

False Lash 101

It took me a while to master the application of false lashes, but once you learn, you'll be hooked! I find that the right lashes not only help to enhance my makeup look, but also help to give me a little confidence boost too. They make a perfect accessory for any special occasion. Here are my tips for finding the perfect style for you, how to apply them and some common mistakes to avoid!

Choosing a lash

Finding the right lash for your eye shape and personal taste is essential. Lashes often get a bad name for being OTT, but there are so many incredible natural lashes out there that don't get as much attention as they deserve (most probably because people can't tell you're wearing them!). If you have smaller eyes or are new to applying lashes, try a pair of three-quarter-length strip lashes. They are much easier to apply and comfortable to wear so make a great starter lash. They also look incredible with a cat eye as they really help to add a feline shape. If you're a little older and think false lashes would look too much on you, try using individual or cluster lashes. They are a much more natural way to add fullness and volume to your lashes and are virtually undetectable to the untrained eye. I personally love Eylure's lashes because they are attached to the packaging by the lashes themselves (rather than glue along the band). This means they don't get misshapen when you remove them from the packaging, making them easier to apply.

Preparation

Preparation is half of the work when it comes to false lashes. Firstly, if you're using strip lashes, you will need to make sure they are the right length for your eye. Remove them from the packaging and place them along your lash line without any glue. You want them to run from about 5 mm away from where your natural lashes start (so they aren't uncomfortable and poking you in the eye!) to the end of your natural lashes.

If they are too long for your eye, cut the required amount off the lash using nail scissors, ensuring you are cutting length from the outer corner of the lashes to keep the tapered shape of the lash on the inner corner intact. Then you want to apply a small amount of glue along the back and top band of the lashes. Wait for it to dry for about forty-five seconds before application. A lot of brands say thirty seconds, but personally it works better for me if you leave it for a few seconds longer for the glue to go tacky.

Application

Once the glue is half-dry, apply them to the lash line, starting at the centre of the eye, making sure the band is as close to your natural lash line as possible. Hold the centre section in place while using your other fingers to push down either end of the false lash to align with your natural lashes. Hold the lashes down for about fifteen to twenty seconds whilst waiting for the glue to dry (don't move at this point – a common mistake that results in your lashes not sticking properly!).

Once the glue is completely dry, gently push the lashes upwards from below, making sure they are sitting correctly along your lash line, opening up your eye and making the most of the added length and volume. Good lash glue should dry completely clear, so don't worry if you can see the glue a little bit; once it's dry you shouldn't be able to see it at all.

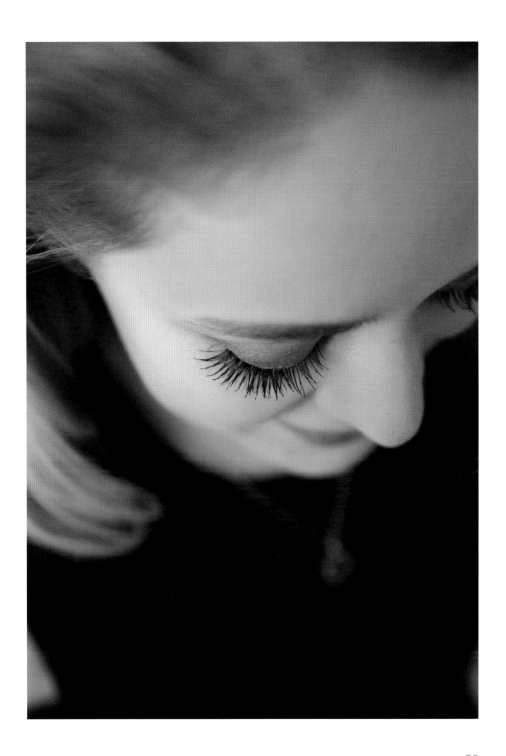

Blending

There a couple of tips and tricks you can use to help blend your lashes into your natural lashes, making them look more realistic. Try using a liquid eyeliner to run a thin line across the back of the lashes, along the natural lash line. This works especially well for three-quarter-length lashes as it helps to continue the line of the band. I also like to apply a little mascara onto the lashes after application to help blend my natural lashes into the falsies. However, if you want to reuse the lashes, I'd recommend skipping this, otherwise you'll have to clean the mascara off them after use, which can be tricky.

A sticky subject

Finding the right glue for your falsies is half the battle! The glue included with lashes is often not very good, so I'd recommend buying a separate tube. My personal favourites are from Duo and Eylure. If you tend to get a bit messy with your glue, you can get dark grey-tinted glue which blends better with eyeliner and mascara. However, it can be slightly less sticky and remember that it dries black rather than clear, so can take practice to master!

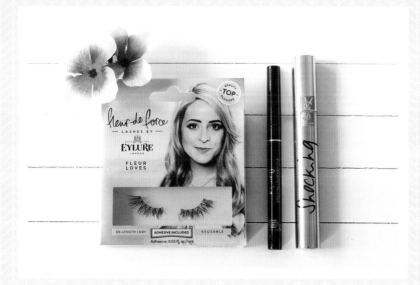

All That Glitters

Ways to Wear Glitter and Still Look Sophisticated!

Like most girls, I love a touch of glitter, but it can be a tricky balance when it comes to pulling off glitter in makeup. Wearing too much or applying it in the wrong way can be a recipe for disaster, but choose the right shade, product and application technique and it can turn any average beauty look into something special and help to highlight your assets.

EYES

When applied well, glitter on the eyes can be most alluring. The first hurdle is finding the right product, as loose glitter can be very messy to wear for an extended period of time. Pressed powders or creams are the most convenient formulas when it comes to glitter eye shadow, with Japanese brand RMK making some of the most impactful and beautiful glitters (a lot of these are limited edition, but they have a few available at any one time). Urban Decay also has a great selection, but some of the heavier glitter shades can have quite a lot of 'fallout' and can be messy if not applied with care. My favourite way to apply these heavier glitters is as a final touch to my eye shadow. This works especially well with a smoky eye. I like to press a little glitter onto the centre of my eyelid using my finger to work the shade into my existing eye shadow.

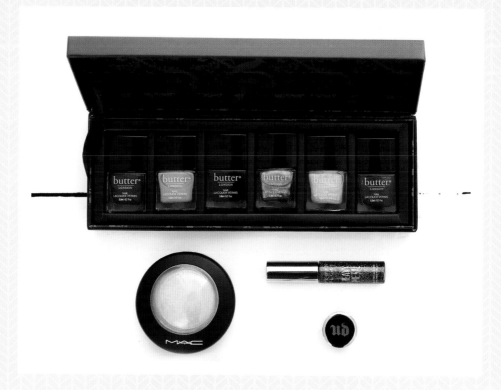

If glitter shadow is a bit much for you, glitter eyeliner is another beautiful way to accentuate your eyes. From the dazzling full-on glitter liquid liners that Urban Decay do so well to much more subtle versions of kohl and gel liners with a hint of shimmer in them, there are several ways you can experiment with this look. Again, many of these liners crop up as limited editions in Christmas makeup collections, but Urban Decay's 24/7 pencil selection offers a few different shimmery shades and By Terry's Terrybly pencils have some great shimmery neutral shades.

LIPS

Glittery or frosted lips are incredibly hard to pull off and I would generally avoid this look unless you're dressing up or at a festival. However, if you do want to go for the glitter-lip look, your best bet is to match the colour of the glitter as closely to your base lipstick as you can, apply a couple of coats of lipstick then pat the glitter on top, concentrating on the centre of the lips to give the illusion of fuller lips.

FACE

Again, proper glitter on the face is a look best reserved for festivals and fancy dress. Instead, choose a finely milled powder highlighter with shimmer in it to achieve a more striking highlighted look that is perfect for special occasions and nights out. My favourite products for this kind of look are MAC's Mineralized Skinfinishes.

NAILS

Nails are definitely one of the easiest places to incorporate a little glitter into your look. Full-on glitter polishes are a favourite of mine, especially at Christmas. My favourite brands for glitter are Butter London and Deborah Lippmann. Accent glitter nails are also a nice way to add a little sparkle to your nails without going all out, but nail trends tend to come and go very quickly and the accent nail isn't really very popular at the moment. Right now I much prefer a subtle shimmer top coat (my favourite being Butter London's iridescent Glad Rags).

Fake Tanning

Glowing-looking skin and a perfectly even tan can really help to pull your look together, especially in the summer months when you're likely to have a little more skin on show. Fake tanning is, however, one of the easiest things to get wrong if you don't take your time and prep your skin properly, and there's nothing worse than the panic of a streaky tan or orange hands when you want to look your best for a special occasion. Here are my top tips for achieving a perfect-looking tan at home with minimal fuss.

Prep your skin

Before even thinking about applying fake tan, you want to make sure your skin is free of any dry, flaky patches that the pigment will cling to. Start by thoroughly exfoliating your whole body the day before you tan (or in the morning if you tan at night). Spending a lot of money on body scrubs is usually not necessary, as they often don't go very far and cheaper alternatives can do an equally good job. My favourites are the ones from Soap & Glory as they are effective, affordable and come in huge tubs so will last longer than the average. The Clinique Sparkle Skin body scrub is also one of the most effective I've tried, but is more expensive. You want to really work your scrub into your skin in circular motions to ensure the best results, and follow this up by rinsing it off and shaving any areas that need it, to give yourself a really smooth canvas for the colour to develop. If you can, it's better to exfoliate for the few days leading up to when you fake tan, to ensure your skin is really even and smooth. If you don't have time for this, one round of exfoliation is better than nothing so if you want your tan to look even and last for longer, don't skip this step! If you wax, make sure you leave about twenty-four hours before tanning, and if it's possible to leave a couple of hours between shaving and fake tanning, then do so. It's best not to apply fake tan to irritated skin.

After exfoliating, you want to make sure you moisturise, concentrating on the drier parts of your skin such as ankles, feet, knees and elbows. There are some specialist pre-tanning lotions on the market (St. Tropez is my favourite); however, if you don't want to invest in these, just look for a normal body lotion that is oil-free. It's best to wait at least a few hours (or overnight) between moisturising and tanning. When you come to apply your fake tan, make sure your skin is free from any deodorant, perfume, makeup or oils.

Choose the right product for you

Choosing the right tanning product for you will depend on how tanned you are already and how tanned you want to go. If you're pale-skinned and want to add just a touch of colour, try a gradual tanner, or a 'light' tan. If you have olive skin, are already tanned or if you want to go darker, use a 'dark' tan. My favourite tanning brand is St. Tropez as it delivers the best colour results for me personally and lasts about five days. I especially love their Express Tan that develops in one to three hours. It's perfect if you don't like the smell of developing fake tan as you can wash it off after just a few hours and still get the same depth of colour. Their tanning oil is also great, especially if you tend to have dry skin. For a more affordable option I would recommend Rimmel's range of fake tans, and for the longest-lasting fake tan (but possibly the most expensive!) I would recommend Vita Liberata.

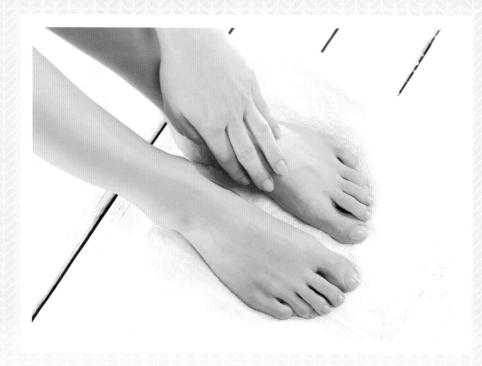

Tip When tanning your face, I would recommend using a product specially formulated for the face, as the skin is more sensitive. My personal favourite is James Read's Overnight Tan Sleep Mask.

Application is key

The best investment you'll make if you want to fake tan is to buy a sponge tanning mitt. These are a couple of pounds from pharmacies or beauty stores and will help ensure an even application, avoid streaks and most importantly you won't get the dreaded orange palms! These can be washed in the sink with hot soapy water, dried and reused (I'd actually recommend doing this after every use to avoid product build-up). I've found that mousse textures are the easiest to apply with a mitt: pump the product directly onto the mitt then work it into your skin in quick, short motions until it's evenly blended, starting from the centre of each area and working outwards. It's advisable to get someone to help with application to your back, unless you've got unnaturally long arms – it's tricky to get it evenly without help!

After you've applied your tan, wait about ten minutes before getting dressed to ensure the tan is completely dry. This will also help to ensure you get the most even results. If your tan isn't as deep as you'd hoped you can build the colour up over two to three days. The best time to tan is usually at night, as your tan will have time to develop without you washing or wearing tight clothing. If you're worried about the tan transferring onto your sheets, simply ensure you're wearing full-length pyjamas and pop a towel on your pillow, or use an old pillow case. Fake tan stains on sheets should wash off with a good stain remover though, so don't worry too much if you do get some on your bed sheets! If you apply fake tan in the daytime, try to avoid wearing tight-fitting clothes that day to ensure your colour develops evenly.

Making your tan last

You've gone to all the effort of achieving a perfect, streak-free, natural-looking tan, now you want to make sure it lasts as long as possible! The best way to do this is to keep your skin moisturised by applying lotion or body butter on a daily basis. Also try to avoid reapplying fake tan when your tan is still fading, as this will lead to colour build-up, which can then look patchy and orange. Instead, go back to the beginning and exfoliate the remaining colour from your skin as best you can before reapplying.

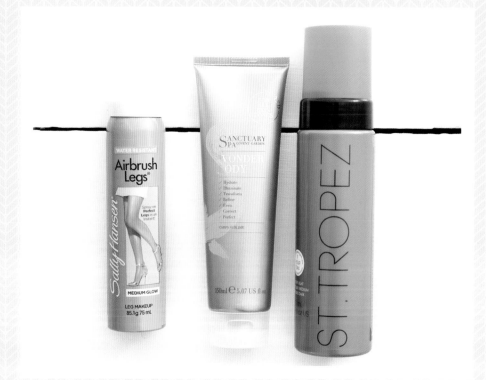

Tip If you get fake tan on your hands, or anywhere you don't want it, try washing it off with toothpaste (yes, toothpaste!) and a soft scrubbing brush, or try mixing baking soda with water to help fade a blotchy tan.

Perfect Party Legs

Perfect party legs take more than just fake tanning – here are my top ten skin-finishing products to get healthy-looking, shimmering skin for special events.

BODY MAKEUP

It might sound a little OTT but body makeup has secured a permanent position in my party-prep product line-up. Different products have varying degrees of coverage, but the right body makeup applied well can make your limbs look totally flawless. My most-used product is Sally Hansen's Airbrush Legs. Perhaps the most well-known body makeup, this has medium-buildable coverage. Its truly water-resistant formula doesn't budge in the rain and will not transfer on to your clothes or your car seat. It only comes off when you want it to (in the shower with the help of hot water and soap). Soap & Glory also make a similar product called Glow Getter, which is slightly more focused on bronzing as well as coverage, so if you haven't had the time to fake tan beforehand, it has you covered. I also rate MAC's Face and Body foundation for adding coverage where required, but I personally prefer using it for the upper body (chest and arms, usually) as it has less coverage and less shimmer than the others.

SKIN-PERFECTING SERUMS

My obsession with skin-'perfecting' serums started with the This Works Perfect Legs Skin Miracle. A product I never realised I wanted or needed, this tinted serum gives your skin a natural sun-kissed glow while being formulated with vitamins C and E for improving any pigmentation, scarring and uneven skin tone. It also has arnica which may help reduce bruising (great if you're clumsy like me!) and smells incredible to boot. The colour is wash-off but the skincare benefits only improve with regular use. It's expensive, but a little goes a long way so one tube will last you for ages. A more affordable alternative is Sanctuary's Wonder Body balm. This has a thicker texture and a slightly more illuminating effect on the skin, but has the same imperfection-minimising effect.

SHIMMERING OILS

Glitter-infused body oils are another great choice when it comes to skin finishing, especially in the summertime as they really help to accentuate sun-kissed skin whilst being intensely moisturising at the same time. My favourites are Nuxe's Huile Prodigieuse OR, which is a shimmering version of the French cult classic multi-use oil, and Estée Lauder's annual summer limited-edition Bronze Goddess body oil, which is scented as well.

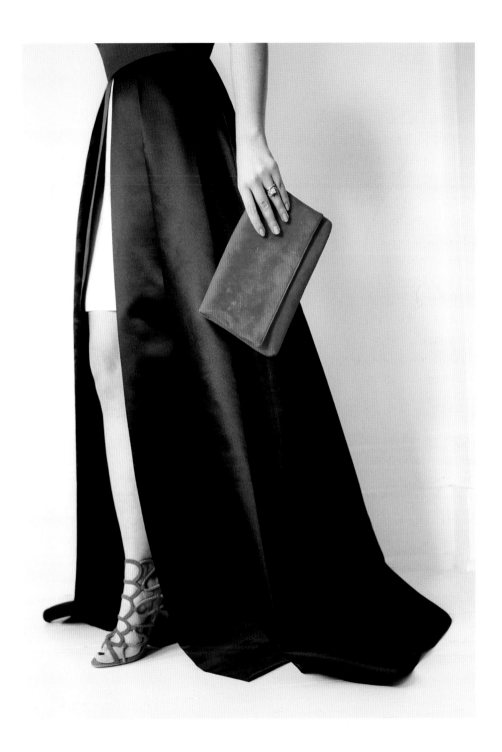

Post-Party Skin Saviours

We spend so much time prepping for events to make sure we look and feel our very best, but we forget about looking after ourselves afterwards. Late nights and lots of makeup combined with plenty of rich food and alcohol can start to take its toll on your skin, so treating it well post-party can help to minimise the effects and keep you looking bright and fresh regardless of how late a night it's been.

Hydrate

The most important thing when it comes to helping your skin renew itself after a big night is to rehydrate. Try to drink water before you go to bed and when you wake up to help minimise dehydration. It might help your hangover, but it will also help to improve the appearance of parched skin, under-eye circles and potential breakouts too.

Treat your skin

No matter how tired you are at the end of the night, try your best to remove your makeup and moisturise before you hit the hay. Micellar water is the quickest and easiest way to get every last scrap of makeup off (my favourites are the Simple one and Bioderma's Sensibio H2O). A rich night-time moisturiser will also help to ensure your skin is in its best shape when you wake up in the morning. I love Fresh's Black Tea Firming Overnight Mask as it makes my skin feel smooth and fresh when I wake up. In the morning it's also worth giving yourself a mini at-home facial. Exfoliate, apply your favourite moisturising mask, an antioxidant serum if you have one and some moisturiser.

Facial massage

Facial massage is a great way to help your skin look its best after a long night. Massaging your products in well is a good opportunity to increase your circulation, reduce puffiness, release tension and help your products to absorb better into the skin. Massage in circular and upwards motions, focusing on the temples, forehead and jaw line. You can do this with both your cleanser and moisturiser, serum or oil.

It's all in the eyes (and lips!)

Your under-eye area and your lips are often the first places to show signs of dehydration, so it's worth applying a decent eye cream to keep bags at bay. Eye gels are marketed as the best products for bags, but I don't find them to be very moisturising at all. I love Indeed Labs' Eysilix eye cream, which is both hydrating and de-puffing at the same time.

My favourite skin-hangover curing products

* Simple micellar water
* Fresh Black Tea Firming Overnight Mask
* Kate Somerville ExfoliKate
* First Aid Beauty Instant Oatmeal Mask
* The Organic Pharmacy Antioxidant Face Cream
* Indeed Labs Eyesilix Instant Eye Rescue
* Palmer's Cocoa Butter lipbalm

7 Party-Beauty Makeup Hacks

★ If you're getting ready in a hurry, use a credit or store card as a mascara shield, placing it behind your lashes as you apply your mascara. This way you can fully coat your lashes in a matter of seconds and not get any mascara on your eyelids in the process. A spoon also works well for this!

★ You can use the same card as a guide to applying neat winged liquid eyeliner in a few seconds by placing it diagonally at the outer corner of your eye and tracing along the edge.

★ When applying under-eye concealer, apply it in a triangle shape (not a curve) under your eye, pointing downwards with the lower lash line forming the shorter side of the triangle. This will help to fully conceal any under-eye circles and make the eyes look brighter and more awake. Always remember to choose an under-eye concealer at least one shade lighter than your foundation.

★ If you're giving yourself a DIY mani but don't have time to wait for it to dry, invest in a decent top coat – Seche Vite is my personal favourite. Quick-dry drops may seem like a gimmick but they really do work (my favourites are from Deborah Lippmann). These two combined will leave your nails dry to the touch in just a few minutes.

★ If you're out and about and notice that your lipstick is bleeding but don't have a lip liner to hand, take it off and prime your lips with concealer before reapplying your colour. This will help to keep the pigments in place and make your lipstick last for longer.

★ If you're taking only a small clutch bag out, try bringing multi-use products with you. Lipstick doubles-up as a blusher and the right shade of matte brown eye shadow can multi-task as a contour for your cheeks, eyes and brows.

★ If you come to apply your makeup and your liquid eyeliner pen has started to dry out, give it a final burst of life by putting it point down (with the lid on) in a cup of hot water for a minute, taking it out, shaking it vigorously and then running the nib back and forth across your hand. This will help to get the product flowing again, even if only temporarily (it's probably time to buy a new one!).

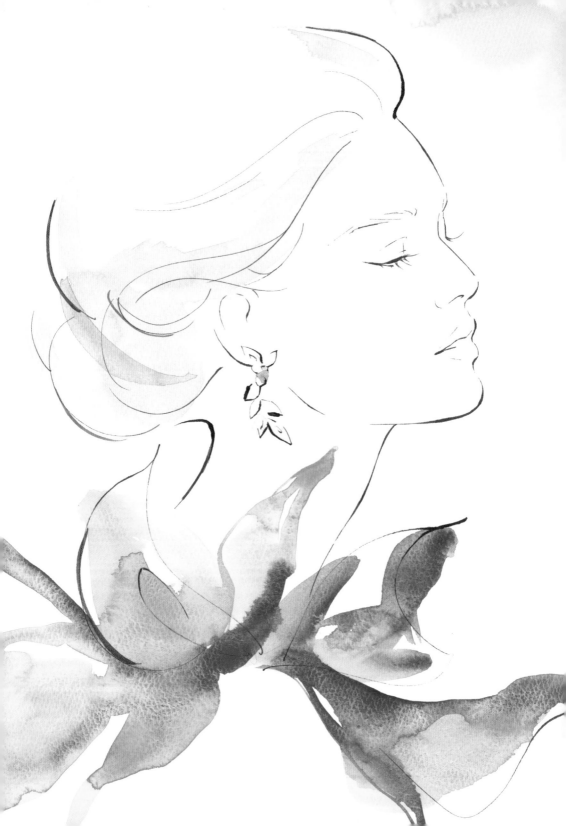

Hollywood Hair

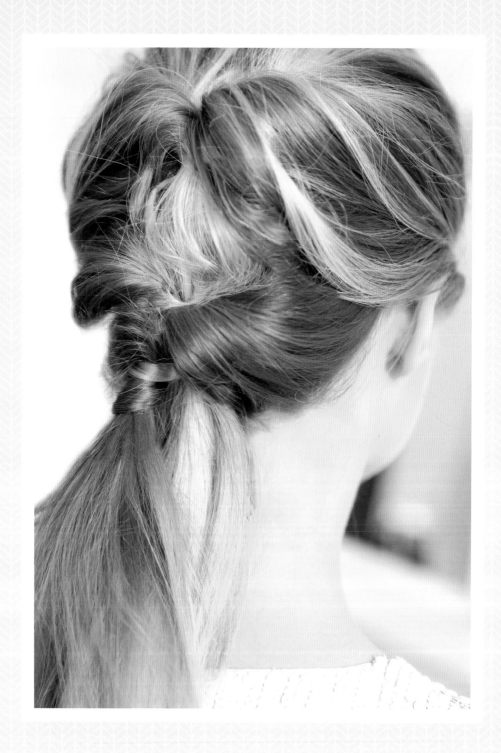

Introduction

When it comes to special occasions, well-styled hair is as important as your makeup for helping you to achieve a perfectly polished look. If you don't have the time, budget or access to a professional stylist for special-event hair, this chapter is designed to help you not only find the right tools to learn to do it yourself and get the best results, but also give you some inspiration for different hairstyles and looks for any occasion. Just remember that, as with makeup, practice makes perfect. If you're planning on doing your own hair for a very special event, it's worth having a couple of practice runs beforehand to save you stress on the day!

5 Perfect Up-Dos You Can Do at Home

THE LOW MILKMAID BRAID

This is a look that I wore in a winter lookbook video this year and I got so many questions asking about how I did it and complimenting the look in general. You can style it down by loosening the plaits and pulling out baby hairs at the front, or smarten it up by leaving the plaits smooth and sleek.

Step 1 Section your hair in half as you would for pigtails. Carefully brush though each half to ensure the roots are smooth. The placement of your parting depends on what you prefer, but I think this style looks really pretty with a centre parting. Neatly plait each side of your hair, starting as high up as you can to get the most dramatic look (preferably with the plaits starting above your ears.)

Step 2 Secure each plait with a clear plastic poly band, then, if you are going for a more distressed look, start to loosen each plait by gently pulling sections of hair from the inner side of each plait outwards. When you've reached the desired thickness and texture for your plaits, spray in a little texturising spray and work it in with your fingers. This will not only give the plaits a more texturised look, but will also help them to stay in place for longer.

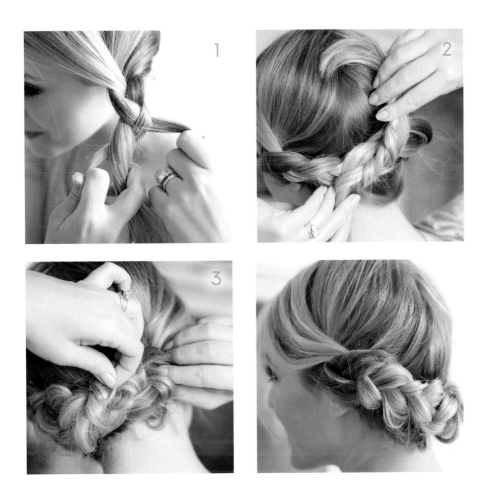

Step 3 Bring one plait around the back of your head and secure it with two bobby pins. Then take the second plait and also run it around the back of your head, along your hairline, tucking the tail of the plait behind the first so you hide the end. Pin it into place with two more bobby pins before securing the remaining length of the plaits with a few more pins.

Step 4 Gently loosen any tight pieces of hair along your hairline for a softer look, then spray your hair with hairspray to help keep it in place.

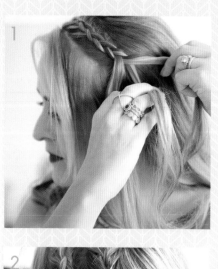

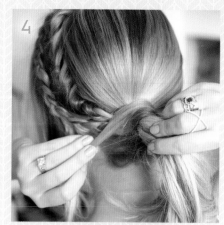

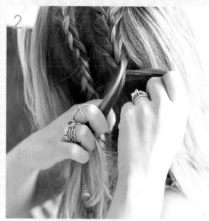

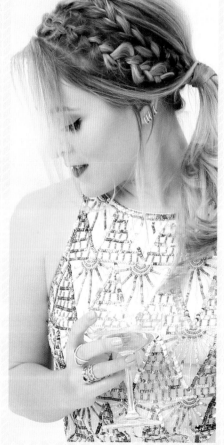

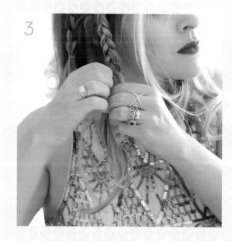

THE DOUBLE-PLAIT PONYTAIL

Continuing my obsession with braids and plaits, this look is a sleek, slightly more formal version of the style of braids I wear a lot. The double layer is much easier to create than it looks, but the Dutch-style braids do take a little time to master, so it's worth practising that before attempting this look. It's a fun, young alternative to a traditional up-do that works really well if you're looking for a sleek, modern look.

Step 1 Take a small diagonal section along your hairline. If you have a side parting, do this on the side of your head with the most hair. Start to French braid this section, working from your parting to your ear. Once this is done, secure it with a clear poly band.

Step 2 Take another similarly sized section of hair just behind your French braid, and braid along the same line, but this time adding new sections to the braid from the underneath, rather than over the top. This is called a Dutch braid rather than a French braid. Again, once you reach your ear, secure the braid with a clear poly band.

Step 3 Gently start to loosen both of the braids by pulling the inner sections out. Repeat this on both braids to both increase their size and give them a more dishevelled look.

Step 4 Finally, brush and smooth the rest of your hair back into a ponytail. You can also backcomb the section around your crown if you like a more voluminous look. Secure it with another clear poly band, then take a small section from your ponytail and wrap it around to conceal the band, tucking the end into the band to secure it into place.

THE SMOOTH SLICKBACK

This is a perfect look for those who don't like to have their hair up, as it gives you the effect of having your hair off your face, but it's still half down at the same time. It's also a great look for modern outfits like tuxedos, jumpsuits and more masculine looks.

Step 1 Brush and straighten your hair (or blow-dry it straight. Separate the very top section of your hair (from about 1–2 cm above your ears, all the way back to your crown) and tie or clip it up out of the way.

Step 2 Take two small sections at each temple from the bottom of the section you've tied up, down an inch, then running all the way back around your head. Brush these sections backward as smoothly as possible and tie them together very tightly into a small ponytail just under your crown using a clear poly band so it's less visible.

Step 3 Take down the top section of hair and backcomb it at the crown, adding texturising spray if you prefer. Then gently smooth the hair backwards to cover the ponytail section. Use hairspray to hold it in place at the front and add some bobby pins at the back section to help keep it in place. Once you're happy with the placement, spray your entire hair well with a strong-hold hairspray to keep it in place. I'd also recommend taking a small bottle out with you in your bag for any on-the-go touch ups!

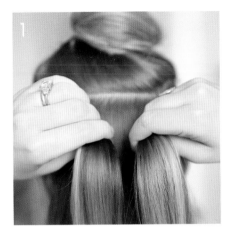

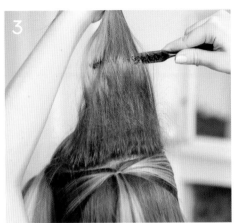

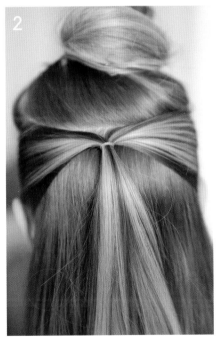

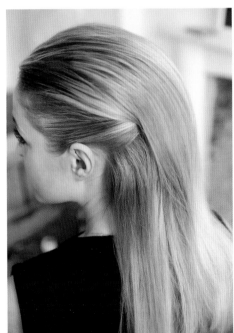

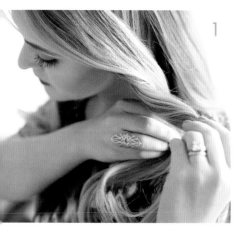

THE TWISTED CROWN

This cute, relaxed-looking twisted crown style is perfect for more boho looks and works best if your hair is already wavy.

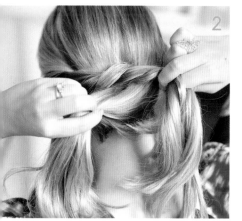

Step 1 Section out two inch-thick sections of hair at one of your temples, and start to twist them around each other. Every second twist, add a little more hair as you go (like you would with a French plait). When you reach the back of your head, secure the twist with a poly band.

Step 2 Repeat this for the other side of your head, then repeat the twisting process on the same-sized sections of hair just below the first twist on each side, so you have two layers of twists.

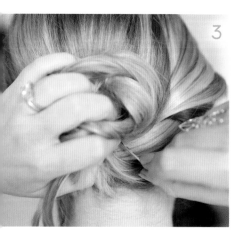

Step 3 Twist the remaining hair around itself and up into a messy bun. Secure with a hairband and a few bobby pins, then use your fingers to loosen up the style around your hairline before spraying with hairspray to help the look stay in for longer.

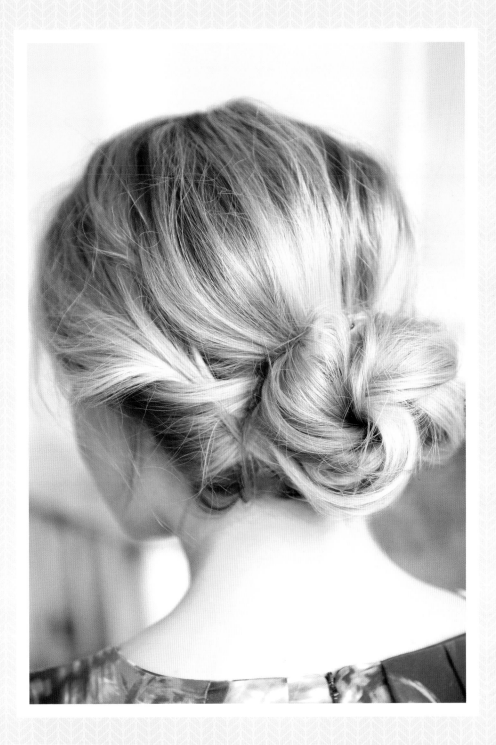

THE TRIPLE-TUCK

This style is the quickest and easiest in this chapter, but it looks awesome! It's an extremely low-maintenance alternative to an 'up-do' that you can wear either as a pony tail, or a sleek chignon at the nape of your neck.

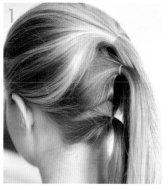

Step 1 Divide your hair horizontally into three equal-sized sections and tie them into three ponytails directly above each other using poly bands.

Step 2 Divide the hair just above each poly band and flip the ponytail over and through this hole. Do this for each ponytail, then tuck the remaining length of each pony through the centre of the next twist.

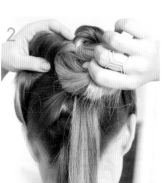
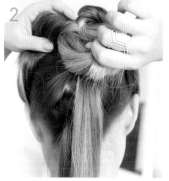

Step 3 You can then either leave the look as a cool, low pony or twist the rest of your hair up into a chic chignon at the base of the neck and secure with bobby pins.

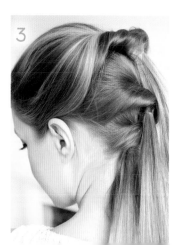

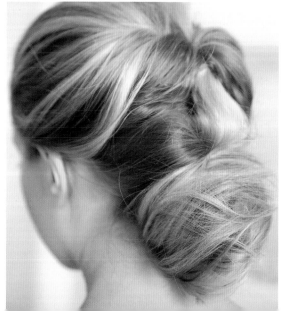

Essential Tools for Creating Occasion Hair

Curling wand

Although you can curl with straighteners, if you want a shortcut to creating the best waves and curls, you'll need a decent wand. The type you choose depends on the type of curl you want to achieve. I personally much prefer wands to tongs, as the lack of a clip on the barrel reduces the likelihood of kinks being created at the ends of each section. My favourite wands are from ghd and José Eber. For more relaxed, beachy waves try a conical wand (the Creative Curl Wand from ghd is great for this) and for bigger, more glamorous curls try a larger-barreled wand like the José Eber 32 mm. For budget options my favourite brand is definitely BaByliss.

Straighteners

If I'm travelling light and have to pack just one heat-styling tool, it's always straighteners as they are the most versatile. Creating different kinds of curls with them takes practice and in my opinion never looks quite as good as when you use a wand or rollers, but it's a good skill to have. The best brand is without a doubt ghd. Despite being a pricey option, their stylers last for years and are the most effective ones I've tried.

Large round brush

A large-barreled round brush is your best friend when it comes to blow-drying your own hair and creating volume and bounce. My personal favourite is one from Goody that has mixed bristles and a ceramic barrel that heats up with the hot air from your hairdryer, reducing drying time and helping to style your hair more effectively.

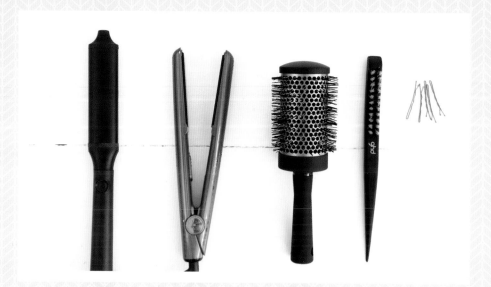

Tail comb

A tail comb is the best way to get really precise partings, whether it's your central parting or dividing sections when styling. They are also great for backcombing your hair to add volume and texture. There's no need to invest in tail combs as you can get great cheap ones from the high street for a couple of pounds.

Poly bands

A fundamental part of my favourite styles and especially so for any braided styles. Clear plastic hair bands are an essential for doing your own hair as they are almost invisible. You can buy them in massive packs on the high street for a few pounds. I never travel without them.

Bobby pins

An obvious one. I'd recommend going for the slightly more expensive matte finish ones as they tend to grip the hair a bit better.

Needle and thread

A much less well-known method of holding hair in place invisibly. My good friend and hairdresser Gareth introduced me to hair sewing on the photoshoot for my last book and it's such a useful little trick to have up your sleeve. It takes practice, but holds the hair so well and allows you to be a lot more creative with your styling than traditional tools.

Top Party-Hair Products - and How to Use Them

Oil and serum

I love hair oils and serums as they are great for injecting some moisture and reducing frizz in my colour-treated hair. I like to use them on both wet and dry hair, but especially on wet hair before blow-drying. They work really well as a detangler as well as a leave-in conditioner and smoothing treatment. They are also a great multi-tasking product to take away on your travels if space is tight, especially if you get one you can use as a body or face oil as well like Elizabeth Arden's Eight Hour All-Over Miracle Oil. My other favourite hair-only options are Pantene's Vitamin E Dry Oil and the classic MoroccanOil.

Styling crème

This is another multi-use product that is a staple of my hair-styling armoury. Crèmes are great as they give you more help with styling than oils and serums because they have some hold. My favourite is again from MoroccanOil. Use them on wet hair for added volume and hold, then on the ends as a finishing serum once your hair is dry.

Texturising spray and dry shampoo

Texturising spray has blown up in popularity over the past few years, but sometimes it's hard to work out the difference between it and dry shampoo, as they are quite similar products. They both contain powders that mattify the hair, but texturising spray usually has more hold than dry shampoo, and dry shampoo tends to be a little more powdery in feel. Dry shampoo is designed to absorb oils at the root of the hair to reduce the need for washing, but the powder also adds texture and body to the hair, so lots of people (myself included) use dry shampoo as a styling product too. My favourite dry shampoos are from Colab and Amika as they absorb oil really well, but are lightweight enough not to be overly drying and cakey, which is really common with dry shampoos. For texturising sprays, my ultimate favourite is Oribe's Dry Texturising spray – but it's so expensive, I only ever buy it occasionally. My favourite high-street alternative is Charles Worthington's Volume and Bounce spray, which has a lot more hold than other sprays, so it's great for up-dos and backcombing.

Hairspray and finishing spray

Another pair of products that go hand-in-hand are hairsprays and finishing sprays. Finishing sprays usually have more of a shine element to them, but most of them have a little hold, too. I would use a traditional hairspray to set more detailed styles, or if you want heat styling to last all day. For more relaxed looks, finishing sprays are often a better option, as they are usually more moveable and touchable. My top recommendations depend on what kind of look you're creating. For very extreme hold for special events, the Bumble & Bumble Classic Hairspray has a strong hold that's still flexible. My all-time favourite all-round hairspray is L'Oreal Elnett because it has great hold but brushes out easily. If your hair is easily affected by humidity, I would also recommend Oribe's Anti-Humidity hairspray. For finishing sprays more focused on the finish than the hold, I love Show's finishing spray, and for a pure-shine finishing spray, I would recommend Bed Head's Headrush (which also smells amazing!).

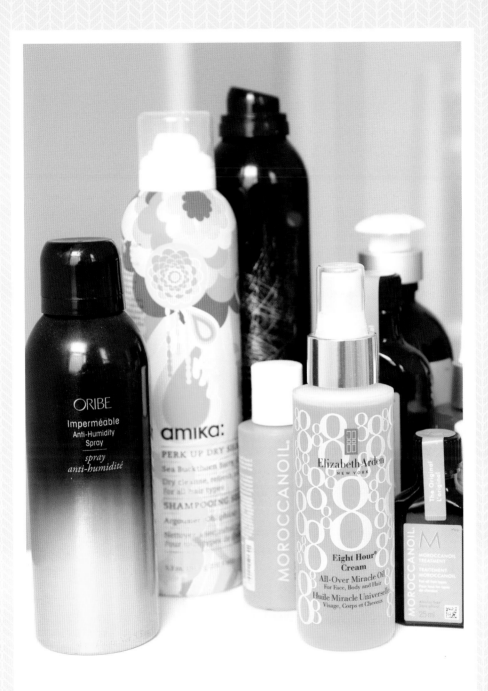

5 Quick Fixes
for Party Hair

There's nothing worse than a hair emergency when you're out and about with no or limited means to fix it, but there are a few hacks and tricks you should know that can prevent these from happening, and will tide you over if you have any major hair dilemmas on a night out. From fixing static to droopy curls, these are my top five quick fixes for party hair.

FIXING STATIC

If you tend to get static flyaways, make sure you work against it before doing your hair for a special occasion. There are several ways to do this: use an intensely moisturising conditioner, use hair oil before blow-drying and don't forget to use hairspray to help hold it in place. If you get static hair a lot, it's also well worth investing in an ionic hairdryer to help combat it – and remember, while hairspray is good at immediately reducing static, over time too much hairspray can actually be quite drying and make the problem worse, so try to combat dryness with treatments and oil to reduce static in the long run. Tumble-dryer sheets are also useful for helping to reduce static caused by your clothes and bed sheets, and you can also line your drawer of hair tools with one (or rest your hairbrush on it) to help minimise static during styling. For on-the-go static reduction, keep a dryer sheet and a mini can of hairspray in your bag, or as a last resort smooth down your style with slightly wet hands, which will help to tame any static and flyaways.

MAKING BOBBY PINS STAY

If you have very shiny, healthy hair, it can be tricky to keep bobby pins from slipping and sliding out of your hair. To prevent this, spray them with a little texturising spray (or hairspray) before inserting them with the bumpy side facing down. Also 'hook' them into your hair for extra grip by inserting them into your hair following the flow of the strands, then flipping them back on themselves into the hair right at the root.

CONCEALING HAIRBANDS

Visible bands or pins are usually not a good look when it comes to occasion hair. Start by choosing a hairband as close as possible in colour to your natural hair, or by using a clear poly band. To conceal hairbands it's really simple to wrap a small section of hair around the band and tuck it into the bottom of the band, but this often slips out and becomes visible. A really neat trick for a more secure way of doing this is to take a large, loose hairpin, and place it (both sides) into the inside of your hairband, in the least visible place, but with the top of the pin still poking out of the hairband. Take a small section of the hair from within the ponytail and wrap it around the band itself. Then take another hairpin and slide all of the hair from your small section into this pin. Push your second pin through the eye of the first pin and remove the second pin entirely, so the section of hair is left inside the eye of the first pin. Finally, pull the first pin down and out of your hair, which will pull the small section neatly down through your band, securing it tightly.

WHEN YOUR CURLS DROP

I get asked a lot by my friends what's my best advice for keeping curls in hair for a full-day event. The truth is, curls will naturally drop out over time (especially if you have thick, heavy hair). Therefore the best thing to do to ensure your curls last is to put the groundwork in to start with when you're styling your hair. Use good styling products (as I said in the previous section, styling creams are great for curls). Always style your hair slightly more curly than you want it to allow for drop out. When you're curling your hair, regardless of whether you're using rollers, a wand or tongs, try to let the curl cool down when it's still curled around something. For rollers, make sure they are completely cool again before removing them, and for tongs and wands, catch the curl in your hand when you remove the wand, keeping it coiled, pin it upon your head to cool before removing it. Never forget to use hairspray, and invest in a miniature bottle of your favourite to keep in your bag.

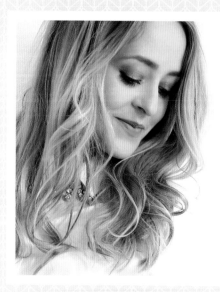

IF YOU GET CAUGHT IN THE RAIN

Getting caught in the rain without an umbrella is a disaster for your hair, and for this reason I would always recommend keeping a compact brush and at least one pin in your handbag. I have a go-to style when it comes to getting caught in the rain that often results in more compliments than my original hairstyle, yet can be created with the help of just one pin!

First of all, get yourself to a bathroom and use the hand dryer to dry what you can of your hair. Then take a small inch-wide section at the front of your head, to one side of your parting (if you have a side parting, take from the side with less hair). Then start to braid this section of hair down to your ear, introducing small sections from along your hairline to the underneath of the braid as you go, creating a Dutch braid. When you reach the nape of your neck, stop adding more sections and finish off the braid as normal. Then take the rest of your hair into a low side ponytail on the other side of your hair. If you have a hairband, secure this now (if you don't, you can still create this look with just one, well-placed, pin!). Take the braid around the back of your head and wrap it around your side ponytail, using the pin to secure the braid into place at the back of the ponytail, so it's less visible. Then smooth the loose side of your hair at the front as much as possible (more help from the hand dryer may be required) and you're ready to go!

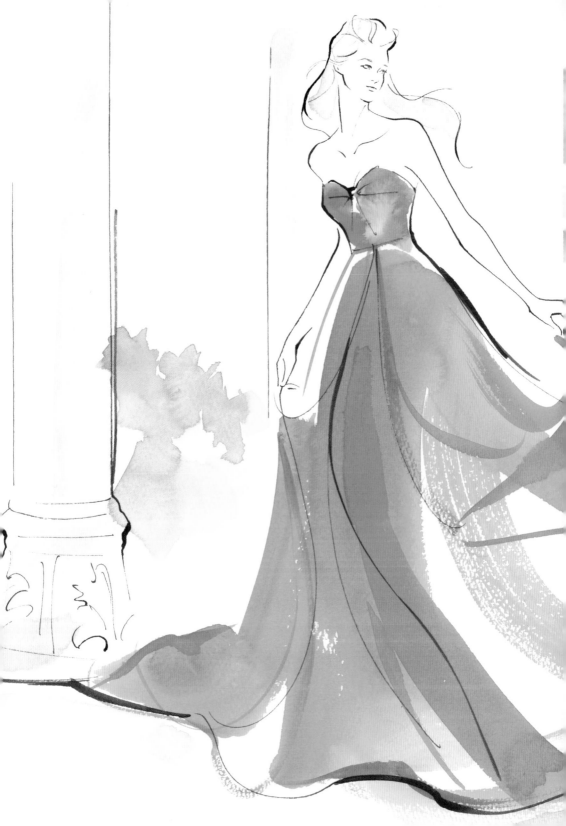

Front-Row
Fashion

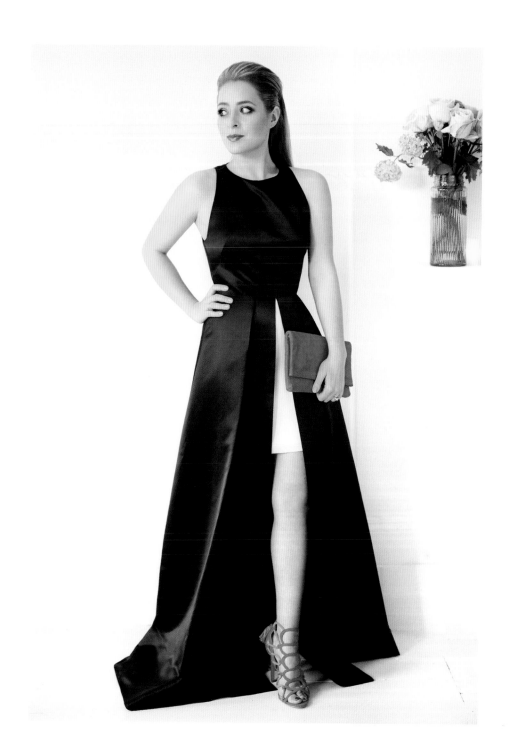

Dresses

Classic Cuts and Shapes You Should Know

When you're choosing an outfit for a special occasion, you want to make sure it's the most flattering for your figure. There are so many different styles and designs out there it can be really confusing and seem like the options are endless! However, it's not as complicated to break down the fashion jargon as you might think. Here are some of the classic dress silhouettes you should know, and the body shapes they suit the most.

The A-line

A-line dresses are generally quite flattering on most body shapes, but especially so for pear-shaped figures and those who want to accentuate the waist while skimming over the belly area. They are generally quite fitted on the top half down to the waist, then the skirt flows out in an 'A' shape.

The Shift

A shift dress comes straight down from your shoulders, skimming over your hips and bum. This type of dress generally looks best on less curvy body types. Generally quite a casual cut, so works very well for daytime events.

The Sheath

A sheath dress is a good alternative to a shift dress if you are a
little more curvy, or if you're looking for something more formal.
They are very similar in shape (both falling in a straight cut from the
shoulders) but sheath dresses are more fitted to the body, often with
darts at the waist to accentuate any curves.

The Shirt Dress

A style that suits most figures, shirt dresses have a structured,
button-up style top half, often with a flowing A-line or skater skirt but
also sometimes with a straight-cut elongated bottom half. They are
great for accentuating or creating the illusion of a defined waist,
while covering the arms and skimming over your belly and bottom
at the same time.

The Drop Waist

Drop-waist dresses can be one of the hardest shapes to pull off
as the lowered waistline creates the illusion of a longer body and
shorter legs. However, if you have a boyish figure and long legs, it
can be a really chic, vintage-looking choice.

The Wrap

A classic wrap dress is another cut that is flattering for most, but
especially so for curvy girls. The wrap and tie detail accentuate the
narrowest part of the waist and the plunging neckline allows you to
show off your cleavage while still retaining a demure look, as wrap
dresses are often a little longer length.

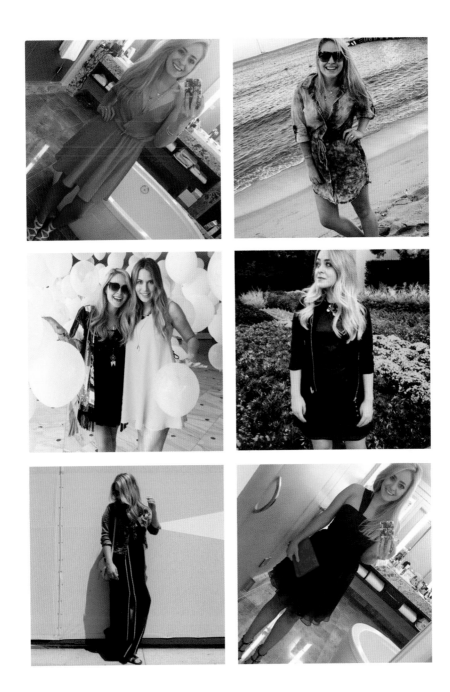

The Empire Line

Another shape that can be tricky to pull off for everyone, but is a good choice for pear-shaped girls. The empire line is fitted around the bust and comes flowing straight down from underneath the bust. This style looks good if you have a small bust and can also be a great choice for disguising a baby bump. It elongates the body and heightens the waist.

The Bodycon

The bodycon dress is one of the most popular modern silhouettes, but can be tricky to wear if you don't have enviable curves or a super-slim figure. If you're apple- or pear-shaped I would advise steering clear of bodycon shapes, but if you do want to go for this all-over tight-fitting shape, make sure you invest in good underwear that will keep the dress looking smooth and clinging to your body in the right way.

The Mermaid

A very formal shape often only seen on the red carpet or in wedding dresses. The mermaid shape is similar to the bodycon in many ways as it is generally tightly fitted from the chest to the knees, but a mermaid dress flows out from the knees to the floor, creating a dramatic curve effect that looks incredible on true hourglass figures.

The Princess

Again a more formal style, princess dresses are characterised by having no clear separation between the skirt and the bodice. They are similar to A-line dresses in shape, but there is no seam at the waist; the material flows directly down. Princess-cut dresses can suit most body shapes if they fit well.

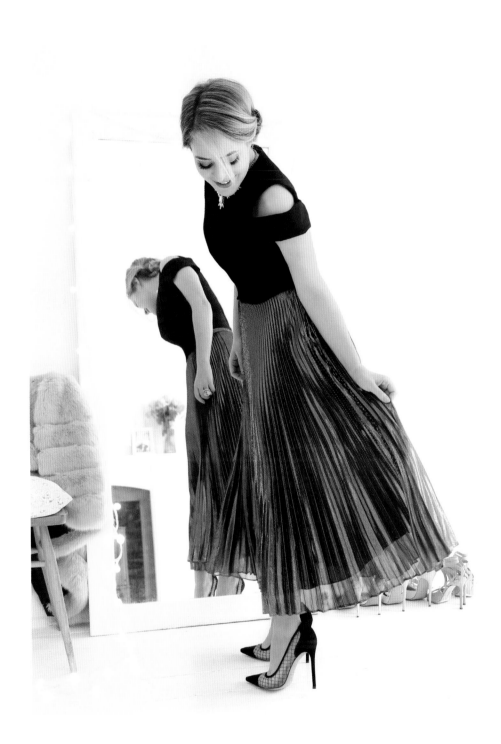

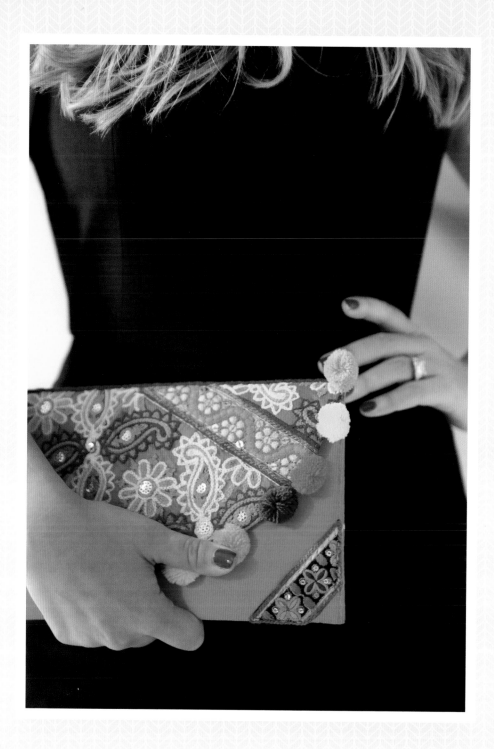

Day-to-Night Fashion Essentials

Whether it's adding a red lip here or a smoky eye there, beauty tends to get more attention when it comes to day-to-night advice. It does, however, really help to think about your wardrobe if you're on the go all day and need to transform your outfit from work-appropriate to an evening look without the opportunity for a full outfit change. There are a couple of things to consider: the first are items that you can dress up or dress down to adapt your look, and the second are smaller items that you can carry with you easily but will instantly transform your appearance for an evening event.

Staple items you can dress up or down

A simple LBD

The ultimate day-to-night staple!

DAY   NIGHT

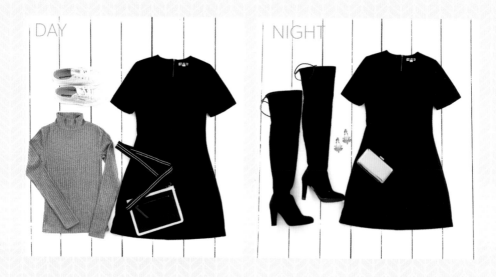

A white shirt

A wardrobe staple that can be worn in the day with a plain skirt, opaque tights and a blazer, or dressed up in the evening by undoing an extra button and adding some jewellery and heels. Just try to pick one that doesn't crease too easily so it won't look tired by the time you've been wearing it all day.

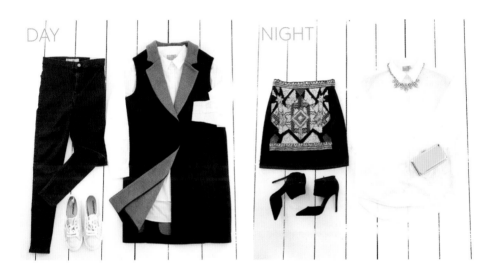

DAY   NIGHT

A classic blazer or leather jacket

Both great daywear staples (depending on the situation) that can be instantly dressed up for the evening with the addition of formal accessories.

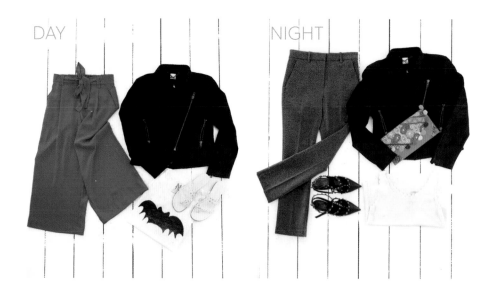

DAY

NIGHT

Leather leggings

One of my personal favourite items for day-to-night transformations.
Leather leggings worn in the day with an oversized jumper and scarf can
be transformed by adding a sleek top and killer heels to achieve a chic,
modern evening look.

DAY   NIGHT

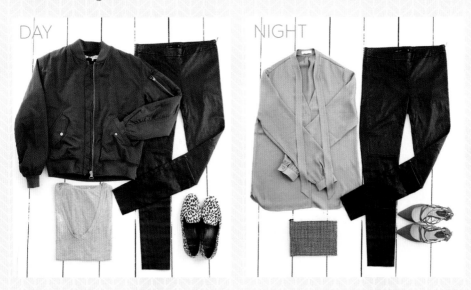

Heeled boots

The perfect footwear for a day-to-night look if you don't have time to change your shoes. Choose a mid-heel so they aren't too uncomfortable to wear all day.

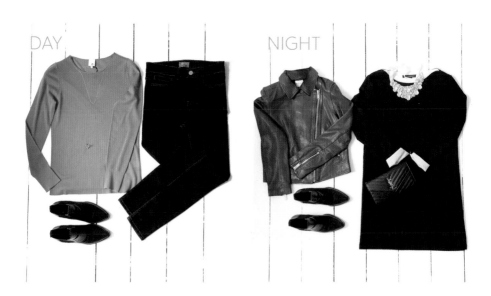

Opaque tights

A great choice for keeping your outfit demure and casual in the day (especially in winter). When it's time to dress up for the evening, you can whip them off and you'll instantly look more dressed up.

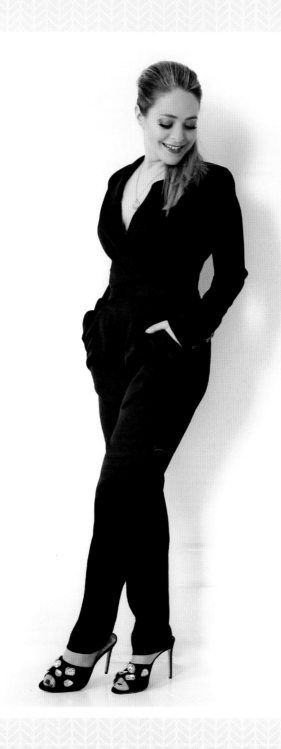

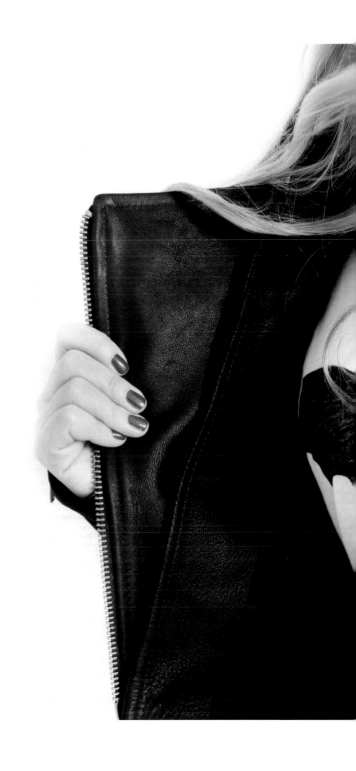

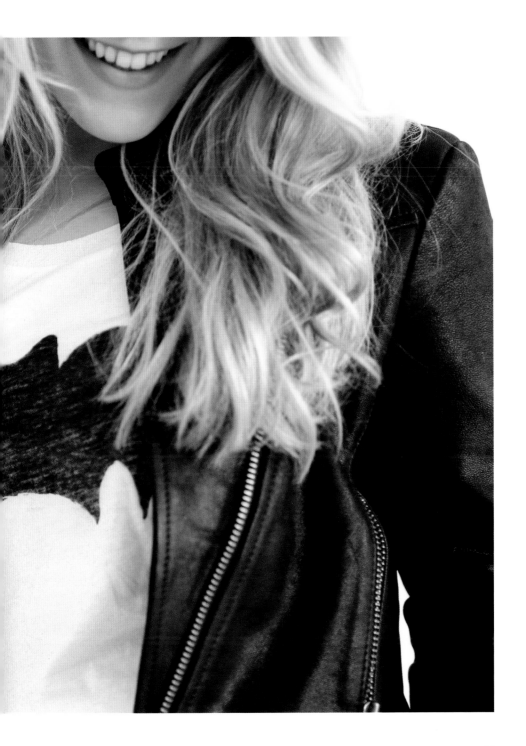

Easy Evening Add-Ons

A skinny belt

The perfect way to cinch in the waist of any loose-fitting top or dress. Choose a metallic or embellished one for a more formal feel.

A simple clutch bag

If you have a small clutch bag that you can fit into your day bag, it's the perfect addition to take you from day to night. I sometimes use a basic clutch as a makeup bag inside my handbag so that I can pull it out and use as a clutch at the drop of a hat if I need to.

Statement jewellery

Another easy way to dress up your look without adding too much extra weight to your handbag. A pair of statement earrings or a necklace can dress up an outfit in an instant.

A silky or sheer shirt

If you can find a sheer or silky shirt that is crease-resistant, it makes a great item to store in your bag and pop on for the evening as it's lightweight and small once folded. Try rolling it up in a piece of tissue paper to protect it and prevent creasing.

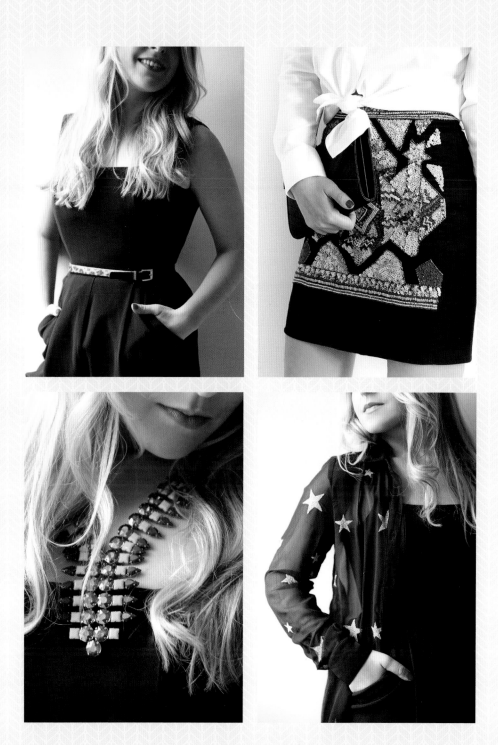

How to Walk in High Heels

When it comes to high heels, my husband always asks me, 'But why did you buy them if they're uncomfortable?!' Let's face it, high heels are simply never going to be the most comfortable shoe in the world, but some are definitely better than others. Finding the perfect ones depends on your individual foot shape. We've all been there – buying a pair of shoes that are just that tiny bit too high, then struggling to walk in them all evening (or simply never wearing them out of the house!). Here are my tips for not only making sure you buy the right heels, but also how to walk in them and how to ensure they stay as comfortable as possible.

Shopping for high heels

When you're trying on a pair of heels, go onto your tip-toes whilst wearing them. You should be able to lift your heels a couple of centimetres off the sole. This determines whether or not you will be able to walk in them properly, as you need that movement in order to avoid tottering around in them. If you struggle walking in heels, always go for a style with a little more support to it. As beautiful as delicate, single-strap sandals look, they have little to no support for your foot and if you're a high-heel newbie, you're very likely to wobble your way through the evening.

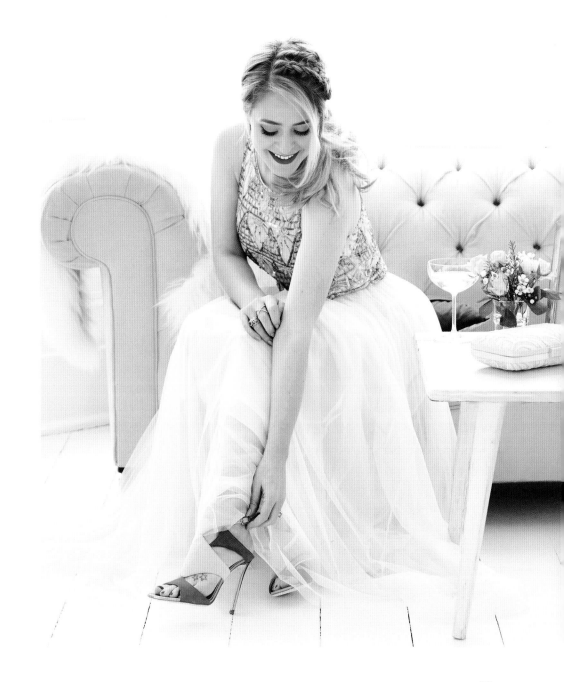

Walking in heels

The most important thing to remember when walking in high heels is to keep your posture as good as possible. Keep your back straight, your head held high and try to avoid looking down at your feet too much. Heels naturally cause your centre of gravity to be pushed forward slightly, which can lead you to hunch over a little bit, giving the opposite effect of the elongated look and sophisticated posture that you want. Take each step at a time. You naturally walk heel to toe, but be wary of putting too much weight on your heels, as you're not as stable in high heels and too much pressure can cause very thin stiletto heels to snap. Keep your core engaged to help with stability. If you can't walk fast in your high heels, it's not a problem as long as you can walk smoothly; just take your time. It helps to swing your hips a little bit with each step but try not to overdo this motion!

Breaking in a pair of shoes

It's never a good idea to wear a brand-new pair of killer heels out for a long evening. If you have the opportunity to break them in a little bit beforehand, then do. You can wear them for a couple of hours at a time around the house, or to shorter evenings out and dinners where you know you're not going to be standing all night. This will give the material a chance to stretch out a little and mould to your feet. If you have a pair of shoes that is just a little too tight, you can take them to a cobbler to have them stretched, or you can do this at home yourself by placing a freezer bag full of water into the shoe and leaving it in the freezer overnight. As the water freezes and expands, it will stretch the shoe a little. You can repeat this until the shoes are sufficiently stretched to the shape of your foot.

Relieving sore feet

If you have sore or blistered feet on a night out, there are a couple of things you can do to help relieve the pain. The first thing is Compeed blister plasters. I always try to have a pack of these in my handbag, regardless of my location or choice of shoe that day. They are simply the best thing for relieving pain from blisters that have already formed and prevent them from getting worse. If you have a pair of shoes that you know rub your feet, take a little pot of Vaseline in your bag. Massage it on any areas that you know tend to rub as it helps to minimise any friction and delay or reduce the likelihood of blisters forming.

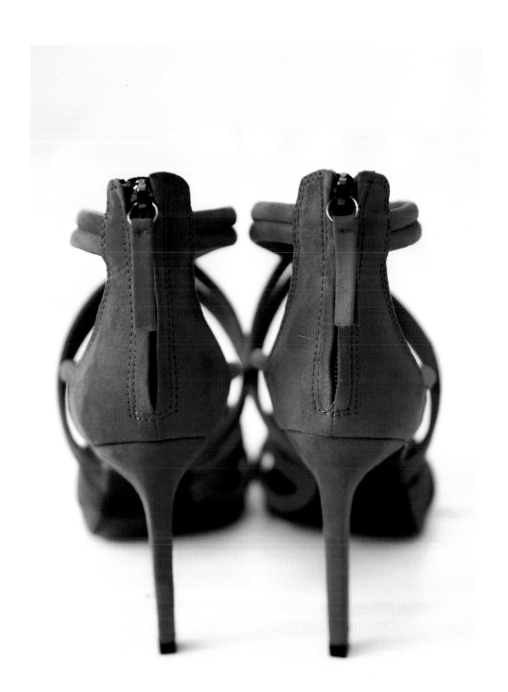

Wardrobe Organisation

Making the Most of Your Clothes

Clearing out and reorganising your wardrobe can be really stressful. It often takes longer than you think and if you don't work out a plan for your new set-up from the get-go, the results might not be what you expected either. However, if you make time to do it properly, the whole process can be really quite therapeutic and organising your clothing makes getting ready in the morning ten times easier! Here are my top tips for decluttering your wardrobe with minimal stress and reorganising it in the best way.

Evaluate the situation

Before you even start pulling things out of your wardrobe or storage space and reorganising it, take a few minutes to evaluate how you currently store your clothing and accessories. Work out how much space you've got to play with and how you can make it work for you more efficiently. This might mean you want to buy some space-saving hanging shelves (Ikea sell very affordable ones) for more storage for your folded items. You can even install a second rail if you want to hang tops and bottoms instead of dresses and it will double your hanging space.

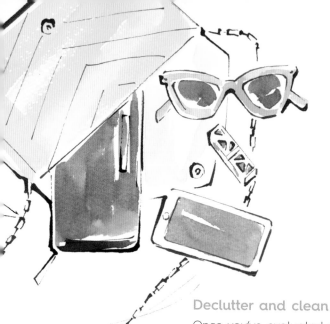

Declutter and clean

Once you've evaluated what space you've got to work with and maximised its potential, you want to move on to the clothing itself. If the task seems a little daunting at first, break it up into sections via clothing type and do one or two categories per day to make it (slightly!) less boring. I work through each type of clothing and divide everything up into three piles: to keep, to donate to charity (or give to friends) and then a 'maybe' pile. Once I've decided what to keep, I fold everything neatly and put it in a pile to one side while I work through all the rest of my clothes. When finished, I return to the 'keep' pile and work out where best to store everything (based on how much of each item I've got!). I also make sure everything is cleaned and wrinkle-free before returning it to the wardrobe, then I go back to the 'maybe' pile and pack everything up into storage boxes, bags or suitcases. I then store these for a season, coming back to them a few months later to reassess whether or not I'll wear them again. Most of the time it's a no and I end up giving it away, but there are always a few things I'm happy to see again and end up reincorporating into my wardrobe!

Organise

When it comes to rehanging your clothes, it's worth investing in decent hangers. My favourites are the velour-finish ones as they are slim so they don't take up a lot of room on your rail, and they are also grippy (unlike wire hangers) so even your slinkier items stay put. Another great tip is to use ring pulls from drinks cans to link together two separate hangers, just don't forget to file down any sharp edges first. You can pair items of clothing you always wear together, or similar items you would always look for at the same time. It also allows you to fit more clothes into your wardrobe.

Try to order your wardrobe in a way that makes sense to you. I don't want to recommend a one-size-fits-all approach for this as what works for some doesn't for others. Arrange your clothing in a way that makes sense for you. I personally like to colour coordinate to some extent, creating a gradient from black to white within each section of my wardrobe. I also like to stack folded clothing in the order that I put items on (from the top to bottom of my wardrobe.) This helps to make choosing an outfit and pairing items together so much easier and quicker in the mornings.

Test it out and reassess

It's worth coming back to your wardrobe a couple of weeks after you've rearranged it to have a think about how your new system is working for you. Tweak it if need be and constantly rearrange. I try to have a full clear-out once a year if I can to ensure I keep on top of things and utilise all the items in my wardrobe to their full potential. My main aim when I'm arranging my clothing is to keep as many items as I can visible, so I don't forget about any items and neglect wearing them.

Curating Your Own Capsule Wardrobe

If you have limited storage space, or want to downsize your wardrobe, the concept of keeping a capsule wardrobe is a great idea. A capsule wardrobe is essentially a smaller encapsulated collection of items that can be paired together in different ways to create a multitude of different looks, while still being diverse enough to cover your bases for all occasions. These are my top five tips for curating the perfect capsule wardrobe that you can update season to season.

Invest in staple items

If you want to strip your wardrobe back to basics, you need to make sure your staple items will last the test of time and look great on you to boot. Learn which cuts and brands fit you the best and stick to them. Don't be scared of investing in good quality staples as they are inevitably the basis of a great capsule wardrobe. Different people's staple items vary depending on what suits them, but it's worth investing in good quality jeans, coat/jacket and boots at the very least. Basics that wear out more quickly (like T-shirts and tank tops) are worth saving money on.

Colour coordinate

An important element of a capsule wardrobe is the fact that all of the items go together. They don't have to be the same or similar colours, but the colours need to coordinate well. Base your choices on your skin tone and colouring as well as your personal taste. There's a whole chapter on choosing the right colours for your skin tone in my first book, *The Glam Guide*. The same tone and colour recommendations apply for choosing your clothing as they do for choosing your makeup.

Dress up and dress down

Try to choose items you know you can dress up and dress down. Dresses that work for the daytime paired with tights and boots, or for the evening when paired with bare legs and high heels are a perfect example. Black skinny jeans, leather jackets and blazers are all also great dress up and down items. You should still try to balance out your wardrobe with a few formal items, but before you buy anything like this consider whether you'll wear it more than once or twice.

Capsule footwear

Your capsule wardrobe can also extend to your footwear and accessories. If you invest in a good pair of high heels, boots and flats you're pretty much covered for all eventualities, but if you also ensure that your choice in footwear is incorporated into your capsule wardrobe, they are the only three pairs you'll need.

Keep your wardrobe visible

Building (and keeping) your capsule wardrobe on a rail, or visible together in one single space, is a great idea as it allows you to construct outfits more easily, encourages you to experiment with new combinations more frequently and ensures you make the most of all of your clothing.

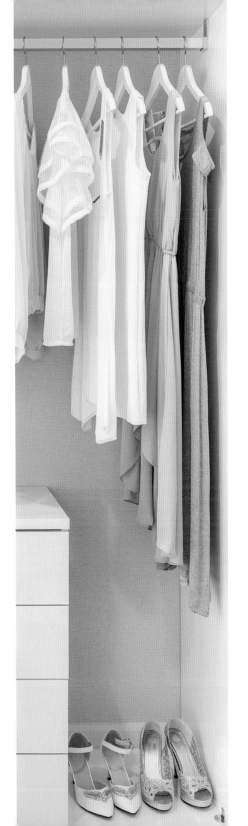

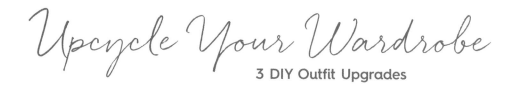

Upcycle Your Wardrobe

3 DIY Outfit Upgrades

You don't have to spend a fortune to update and upgrade your clothing. With a little time and effort, you can update garments you don't use much or love any more to add something new to your wardrobe. I personally love making and customising my own clothing (it's something I used to do constantly as a teenager) so I always like to have a little upcycling project on the go. Below are my favourite three.

DISTRESSING YOUR OWN DENIM

Pre-distressed denim can be more expensive that plain denim due to the amount of work that goes into distressing the fabric, and cheaper versions of 'lived-in' jeans often don't look that great, so it's a good idea to distress your own denim. That way you can decide where and how much detail you want. You can also position the rips or wear to look more flattering on your figure.

You will need

* A pair of jeans (old or new)
* A pen
* A thick glossy magazine
* Razor blades (A Stanley knife or scissors will also work)
* Rough-grain sandpaper

Step 1 Put your jeans on and work out where you would like the distressed sections to be. It looks better if you place the distress where it would naturally happen (on the knees, front and back pockets, end of the legs, on the seams, etc). Mark these areas with your pen so you can place the holes accurately.

Step 2 Take your jeans off and place your glossy magazine inside the jeans behind where you want to start making your cuts to protect the other side of the jean leg and also your work surface!

Step 3 Being very careful, start making cuts with your razor blade or knife, working horizontally across the leg of the jean or pocket. You want to make sure your cuts are at least 1 cm apart at a minimum. It looks good if you make your cuts different lengths to give a bit of variation to the holes (otherwise they can end up looking like a big square). On the pockets and seams you can make smaller, more haphazard cuts to emulate natural distress. Have fun with it, but try not to overdo it or you'll end up with jeans looking like they belong in an early noughties boyband!

Step 4 To refine the look a little bit, take a sheet of sandpaper and rub it harshly over the surface of any areas you want to lightly distress and fade. This works really well on the outer thighs below the pockets.

Step 5 Once you're happy with your cuts, wash and tumble dry your jeans two or three times to really loosen and break up the fabric between your cuts and give the distress a more lived-in look.

Tip For skinny jeans, try cutting off the bottoms of the legs at the ankle bone for a flattering length. When you wash them, the threads will naturally loosen and soften the edge.

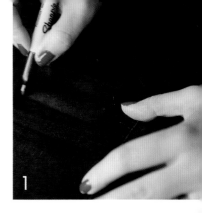

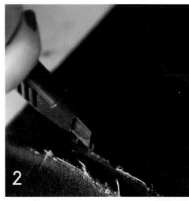

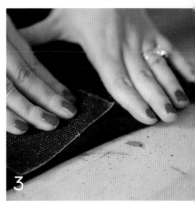

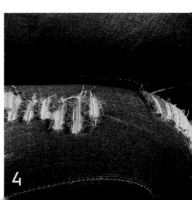

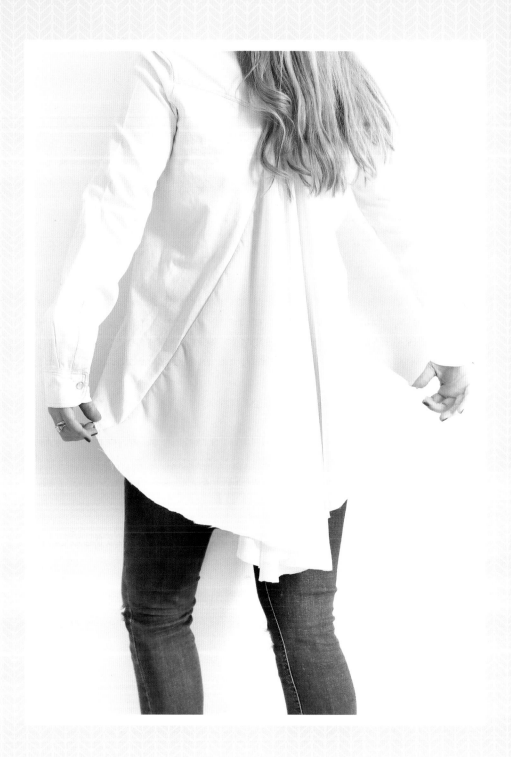

DIY LAYERED-BACK SHIRT

This is one of my favourite DIY fashion projects for updating any simple cotton shirt. The flowing detail on the back adds a feminine touch, so it works really nicely with oversized cuts and men's shirts. If you don't already have one in your wardrobe that you're willing to cut up, you can usually find one at a charity shop, or use one your boyfriend or dad doesn't want any more (I'd advise asking first!). If all else fails, you can pick up a cheap one in a shop.

You will need
* An old shirt
* A metre of fabric of your choice (sheer fabrics work really well for this)
* A sewing machine and someone who knows how to use it if you don't (you can do this by hand but it won't look as good!)

Step 1 Cut a straight line up the centre of the back of your shirt from the very bottom to the seam at the shoulder blades. You can then hem the edges to make it look more professional by folding the raw edge inwards on itself and sewing it up (this is made a lot easier if you iron the edge down before you sew it).

Step 2 Cut a semicircle out of your sheer fabric. The long flat edge should be exactly double the length of the cut you've made down the back of your shirt.

Step 3 Sew your sheer fabric into the back of the shirt.

Tip: You can hem the bottom of the sheer fabric for a neater look, but I personally prefer it with a raw edge.

DIY EMBELLISHED BIKINI

This little DIY project is a simple, quick summer update and you can use your imagination to get creative and design your own look. I love using mini pom-poms for a fun summer festival feel, but you can use any kind of embellishment you wish! If you take a trip to a craft store, you're bound to find something you like.

You will need:

★ A plain string bikini
★ A range of embellishments (pom-pom strings, sequin ribbons etc)
★ A needle and thread in a colour that blends in with your chosen embellishments

Step 1 Lay your embellishments onto your bikini to work out what design you would like.

Step 2 Cut your embellishments to the right length and pin them into place.

Step 3 Take your needle and thread and hand-stitch them onto your bikini and you're done! Extremely simple, incredibly quick and super cute!

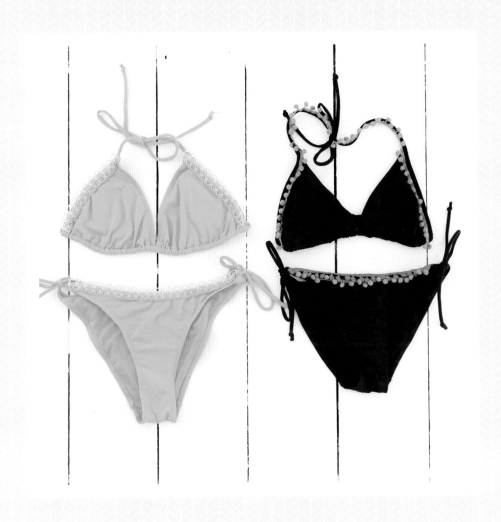

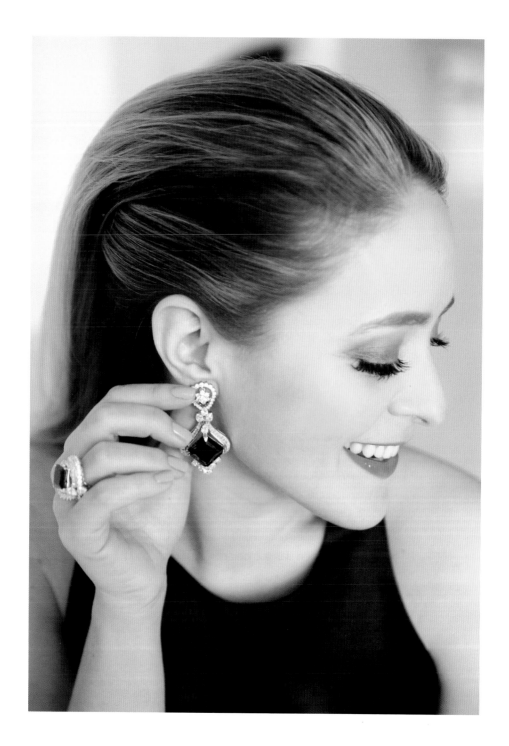

Jewellery Cleaning and Storage Tips

Taking good care of your jewellery will help it age better, but also ensure it stays as bright and eye-catching as the day you bought it. Different metals and stones require different care, so here's a quick rundown of how to care for your precious items.

Silver

Silver tarnishes very easily over time and this process is accelerated by exposure to the air and chemicals, but also by not being worn for a long time, as when the metal rubs against your skin it automatically acts as a tarnish-prevention measure. Silver is very easy to clean up and the quickest way to remove tarnish is by polishing it with a cloth that's been pre-impregnated with silver polish (you can pick them up in supermarkets). If you want to help prevent your silver from tarnishing when it's not being worn, try storing it in an airtight container like a ziplock bag or Tupperware box out the way of direct sunlight, heat, chemicals or humidity.

Gold and gemstones

For gold or white-gold jewellery set with stones, try washing it in a mixture of half hot water, half soda water and a little dish soap. I usually do this in a mug. Leave it to soak for five minutes before swilling it around, then using a soft-bristled toothbrush, clean between the stone and in any smaller crevices. Finally, rinse in cold water and dry off with a tea towel. One of the best investments I've made for helping to care for my jewellery over the past few years, however, has been a sonic jewellery cleaner. This works using the same technology as sonic toothbrushes, vibrating extremely quickly and helping to dislodge dirt and debris from scratches and behind tiny settings that you can't reach with a toothbrush. This works especially well for pieces with lots of tiny stones or intricate detail. Your jewellery looks like new when it comes out and you can pick them up for about £20 online.

Pearls

Pearls can be trickier to clean, as they are very delicate and easily worn down and damaged. It's important that if you do invest in a sonic jewellery cleaner that you don't put your pearls in it, as this will wear them down extremely quickly. A good technique for cleaning pearls is to brush them. Mix up a little baby shampoo with some warm water then, using a large eye shadow blending brush, work your soap mixture onto the surface of the pearls. Finally, wipe any excess shampoo off with a soft, damp cloth and leave the pearls to air-dry naturally.

Costume jewellery

Costume jewellery can also be tricky to clean, as many cheaper metals tarnish very easily and if they are gold- or silver-plated, the plating can wear off if you try to polish it. For very delicate items you can try cleaning them dry, using a combination of a soft-bristled toothbrush to remove any surface dirt, a toothpick to get into any smaller spaces in which dirt may have accumulated and finally a soft cloth to polish the surface. If the piece needs a deeper clean, dip your soft toothbrush in a mixture of soap and warm water then use the brush to clean it. This avoids submerging the piece in water, which may damage it. You can then use a damp cloth to wipe away any excess soap or quickly hold it under cold running water before drying it off with a soft cloth. Don't apply too much pressure as this may remove the plating.

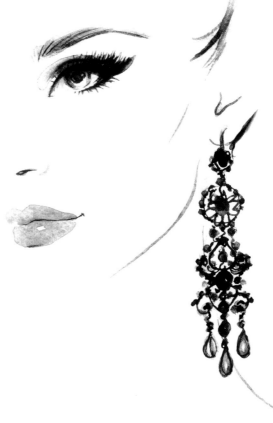

Travelling with jewellery

Looking after your jewellery when you're travelling is really important for preventing damage, tarnishing and dirt accumulation. I like to separate my pieces based on what they are made of and how delicate they are, but it's also worth try out some of the tricks below to keep your jewellery organised, clean and secure while travelling.

★ Keep the soft storage pouches some jewellery comes in, or even the soft cases that come with more premium makeup items. You can then store individual pieces in these for travel. The material can also double up as a polishing cloth too!

★ Use plastic drinking straws to store your necklaces. Run one side of the chain or string through the straw and secure the clasp, this way your necklaces won't get tangled together or damaged.

★ Use spare buttons to store earrings while travelling: thread the backs of the earrings through the holes in the middle of the buttons. This will keep them organised in pairs and make them harder to lose.

★ Use a pill case to store rings, earrings or more delicate items. This stops them from getting mixed up and tangled together, but it's also compact and travel-friendly unlike a lot of the specialist jewellery cases on the market.

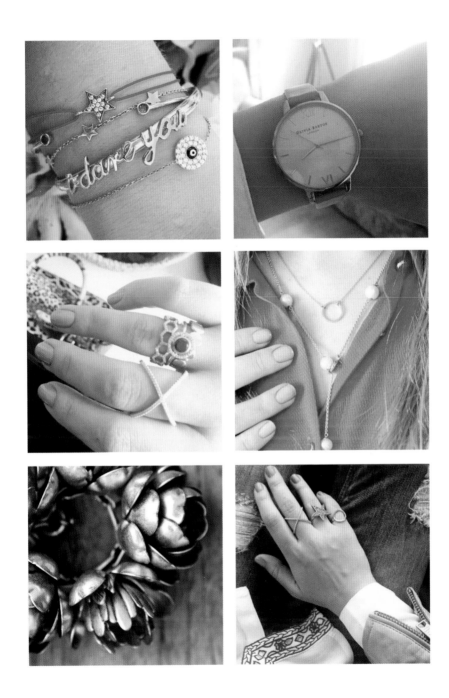

Life-Saving Fashion Hacks

The internet is awash with 'life-saving' hacks at the moment, but some of them are more than a little far-fetched and many of them work in principle but are simply unrealistic for day-to-day life. Below are my favourite fashion hacks that I actually use.

★ Use lemon juice and baking soda to remove sweat stains on white shirts: Cut a lemon in half and rub the juice into any affected areas. Then make a paste of baking soda and water and rub that onto the area too. Wait for it to completely dry before washing the shirt as normal.

★ Use baby powder or cornstarch to remove oil stains: If you spill oil on fabric or leather, heap on some cornstarch or baby powder over the area in question. Leave it to absorb for a few hours before dusting it off into the bin. If it's clothing you can then wash it as normal.

★ Use a razor to remove bobbles from your knitwear: If you have a piece of knitwear that's gone bobbly, use a new razor to very gently shave over the surface layer to remove them.

★ Use hairspray to prevent laddering your tights: We've all heard of using hairspray to stop ladders in your tights getting worse, but if you spray your tights with hairspray when you first put them on at the beginning of the day, it will help to prevent ladders from happening in the first place!

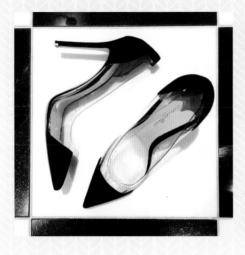
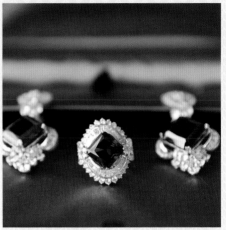

★ Use moisturiser as a replacement for shoe polish: If you don't have any shoe polish hand, you can use a tiny bit of moisturiser to smooth over scratches in leather shoes and accessories. Use less than you think you'll need to start off with and build it up for best results. Start by using a tiny pinprick amount!

★ Use sandpaper to add grip to the soles of your shoes: If you have a pair of shoes that are slippy or unstable, use a very rough-grain sandpaper to add texture to the bottom and increase the grip.

★ Use a safety pin to turn your bra into a racer back: Loop each side of a safety pin around your bra straps on your back to pull them together and turn them in to a racer back. This will avoid leaving your bra visible in racer backtops and save you having to buy a specially shaped bra if you don't wear racer backs very often.

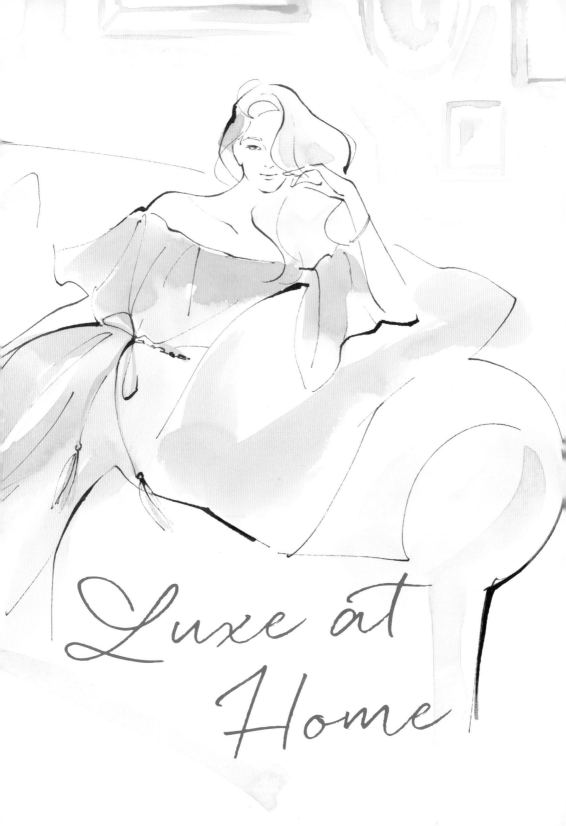

Luxe at Home

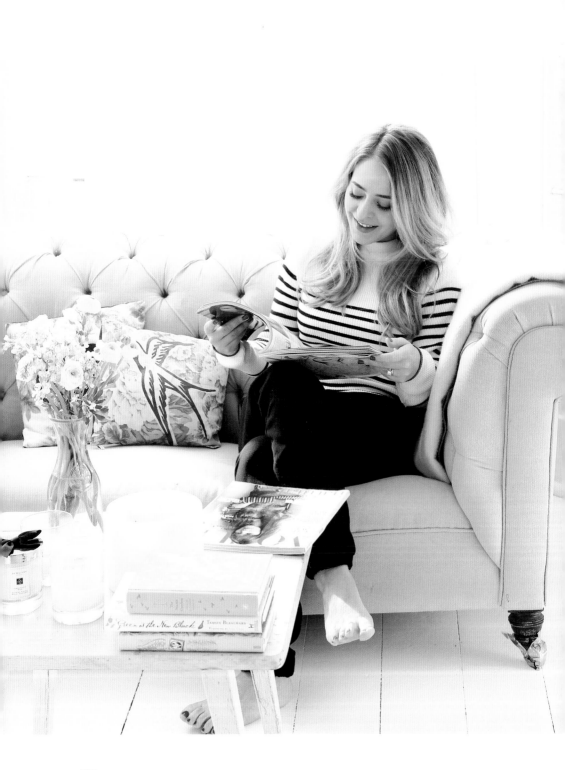

Home Decor
Knowing Where to Start

Nothing makes me feel more relaxed and happy than when I'm living (and working, in my case!) in an environment I love. Whether you've just moved into your first house, recently relocated or you're looking at renovating your home, decorating is exciting but can be daunting at the same time. There are few things, however, that are as rewarding as realising your home decor dreams, being truly happy with the results and creating your own little sanctuary.

There are so many sources of home inspiration and so much choice out there, it can be tricky to make your mind up and decide what style you want to go for, let alone get it right every time! Getting it wrong and having to rethink mid-project is also something you want to avoid, as it's an expensive, disruptive and time-intensive process and in an ideal world you want to get it right first time, every time. So how do you work out what you want to change or decide what style you want to go for? Here are my tips.

Be organised

Before you're even looking at starting a home décor project, do your research and be organised. Setting up a Pinterest board is a great start as it allows you to find inspiration and organise images in a way that is easier to refer back to, and to compare items or styles you're deliberating over. If you're on a budget, be prepared to spend some time researching and trawling the internet for the best value and quality items. You'd be surprised what a few extra hours spent on Google can save you! Try to be patient and consider more expensive purchases over a longer period of time so you can be sure you really want to invest, and to ensure that it will fit in with the rest of your decor. Once I've decided on the style or look I'm going for, I find it easiest to find one piece I really love and build all of the other design around that.

Another important aspect of the planning and organisation process is setting a budget. If you don't set a budget at the start, it's very easy to get carried away and end up with a big bill at the end you weren't entirely prepared for!

Pay attention to tone

It's hard to know how everything's going to look together, especially if you're ordering online or in a showroom with different lighting to your home. Try to get samples of any materials or paints you're ordering so you can compare them in your own environment and check they go together well. It's really important to consider tone when you're choosing colours (be it paint, carpet, tiles, curtains, bedding etc). Decide if you want to go for a cool tone or a warm tone and try to avoid anything that is too different in tone being placed next to each other. If you're choosing paint colours, try painting separate A4 sheets of paper in the shades you're considering. This way, you can easily move them around the room to see them in different lights and locations, and the white background will enable you to see the true colour of the paint better (rather than being tainted by the existing paint or wallpaper on your walls).

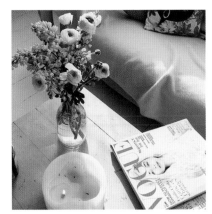
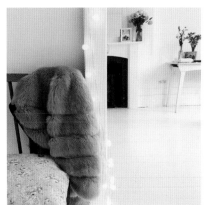
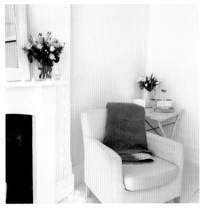
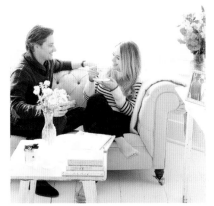
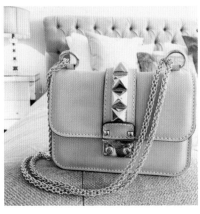
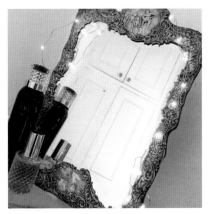

Focus on the bare bones

Once you've got the basis of the room right, then you can focus on perfecting the finer details. It's good to have an image in your mind of the finished result and, as tempting as it is to buy throw cushions, candles and picture frames at the get-go, you won't really know what you need or want in the room until the bare bones are in place. Also bear in mind that every room looks different when you're taking an inspiration image into reality: it might not turn out exactly as you expect, but it might be even better!

Know which corners to cut

Renovating or redecorating your home can be expensive so most people understandably like to cut corners where possible in order to save money. This is totally fine but just think carefully about which corners are worth cutting. Sometimes going for the cheaper option will not work out to be the most cost-effective in the long run (something I learned first-hand when it comes to bathrooms!) but in other cases, it's well worth saving yourself a few pennies and doing things yourself or going for the cheaper alternative. This is often the case with paint colour matching: if an expensive brand has the colour you like, get a paint shop to match it for you using a cheaper brand (usually for half the price!).

Know your limits

We all have our limits when it comes to DIY. The more experienced and crafty you are dictates how much DIY you should be willing to do to get the job done to a standard you're happy with. Doing a lot of the work yourself will help you save heaps of money, but refer back to my first point and be organised: educate yourself about the task at hand as much as possible before undertaking any bigger projects. Whether it's wallpaper stripping, laying tiles or even making curtains, you have to work out if it's something you're confident doing yourself at the risk of potentially ruining any materials you might have paid for. Sometimes it's just not worth it, on other occasions it can save you a fortune.

Be patient

This is the most important tip when it comes to anything DIY, and one I'm personally terrible at! Luckily, my husband is the most patient man in the world, so we balance out quite nicely! Be patient when it comes to making big purchases, deciding when to start bigger home renovation projects and choosing the right contractors to help you. As I previously mentioned, planning carefully with a budget and working out what you can afford if essential. If you can't afford what you want at that exact moment, decide what you can live with for the time being and save until you can realise your dream vision for your home.

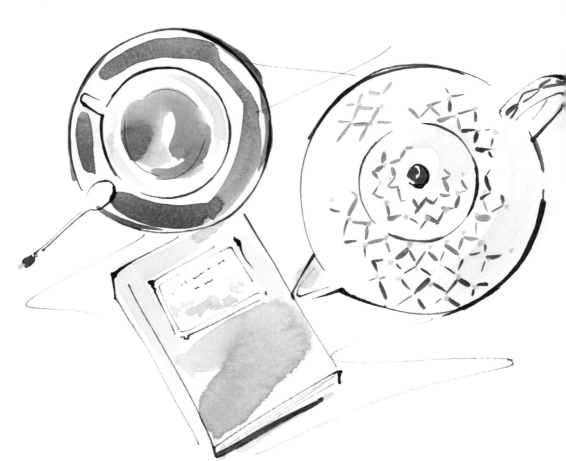

Learning To Declutter Your Life

Your home and especially your bedroom (and work space if you work from home) should feel like your sanctuary. A space where you can really relax and be your most calm, happy self. If you don't currently feel this way about your space then it might be time for a clear-out and a rethink of how you store things. A clear, clean and decluttered space can make a surprising difference to how you feel, function and even sleep.

When it comes to having a clear-out, be it in your bathroom, wardrobe or home office, you need to start by making a lot of mess. Pull everything out from your existing space and have a think about how you can improve the way you store things. Once you've decided on your new storage layout, attack the task at hand in categories. If it's clothing, organise by type of item (tops, scarves, bags) and decide what you really need in your life. If you haven't worn something in over a year and it doesn't have any sentimental value or special significance, it's probably time to let it go. Be brutal! That dress you bought in a sale three years ago because it was an ahhhh-mazing bargain, but you've never worn, is probably never going to be worn.

I bag up all low-value items and pass them on to friends, family or charity shops. Anything more expensive I either put into storage for future generations or sell it on eBay or via a designer re-sale site. If you're on the fence about a few items, the best thing to do is to pack them away in the attic or back of your wardrobe for a few months, then bring them back out the next season, see how you feel about them and make a final decision. Think about what you actually wear the most and focus on that. You should wear at least half of your wardrobe on a semi-regular basis. Occasion wear and sentimental items are different, but you don't need a whole wardrobe full of clothes you never wear.

I organise my clothing by type, but also by colour so that everything is easier to find. The best way to ensure you use everything in your wardrobe is to try to lay out your clothing so you can actually see everything. This way items don't go forgotten and unworn at the back of a drawer or rail.

Clearing out your space can take some time, so be prepared to take breaks so you don't get too frustrated with it. I like to spend different days on different types of clothing, so I don't have to spend an entire day at it. Trust me, once you've finished it will feel amazing! When my wardrobe is organised, I'm automatically more efficient and productive when I'm at home and I put together better, more varied outfits because I'm able to see more of my options together.

TIPS FOR MAXIMISING YOUR STORAGE SPACE

⭐ When it comes to organising jewellery, try investing in clear storage boxes if you have a lot (mine are from Muji). Small, old-fashioned jewellery boxes are pretty but aren't the best way to make the most of your collection. If you can see it, it's more likely to get worn.

⭐ Throw away any bulky hangers as they take up so much space. If you want to go all out, get matching hangers – it looks neat and tidy. My favourites are the slim non-slip hangers that you can pick up in big packs. I get mine from TKMaxx. The copper wire hangers that are everywhere at the moment look awesome but they aren't very practical as items easily slip off and end up at the bottom of your wardrobe.

⭐ Make a feature of your storage. Tall, thin bookshelves are a great storage solution as you can store lots on them and make it look nice at the same time. You can use every other shelf for books, then stack trinkets, picture frames and any other frequently used items on the shelves in between.

⭐ If you have built-in wardrobes, or a walk-in wardrobe or closet, try adding more narrowly spaced shelves (especially in the vertical space above eye level, where the shelves tend to be wider). This will enable you to keep your possessions better organised and often allow you to store more.

⭐ Add hooks to the back of your wardrobe doors. You can use these to store scarves, belts, jewellery or coats and free up space.

⭐ When choosing bedside tables, opt for ones with drawers to help keep the table top clear and also to add more storage to your bedroom, which you can use for underwear, swimwear, jewellery or accessories.

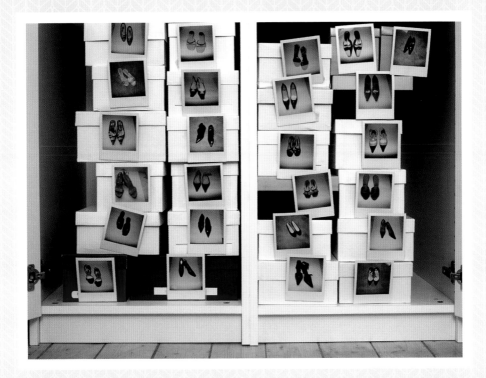

★ If you have space on a wall either in your bedroom or wardrobe, you can use single, slim bathroom towel rails running down the whole wall to create a feature shoe rack for your high heels.

★ Shoeboxes might look nice stacked together, but they aren't making the most of your space. If you can't bear to throw them out, try taking a Polaroid of each style and sticking it to the outside of the box so you don't forget to wear them when you're putting your outfit together in the morning!

★ Create super-cheap yet stylish shelves using small wooden crates. Mount old antique crates on the wall for a shabby chic look, or newer ones for a neat Scandinavian vibe. They are a great way to make a feature of your storage and create two shelf levels.

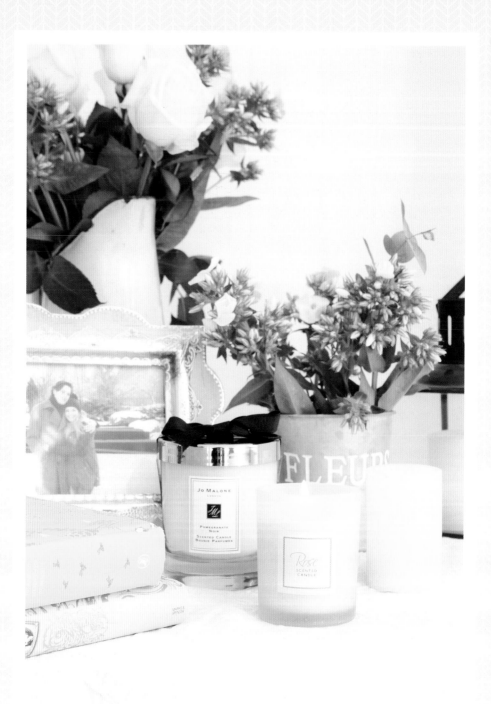

Scenting Your Home

Scented candles are one of my favourite instant updates when it comes to the home, but they can be really expensive. Here are my tips for making the most of your scented candles and my recommendations for the very best candles on any budget.

CANDLE 101

The first burn

One of the most important things to know when it comes to burning a new candle is to allow yourself enough time for the candle wax to completely melt all the way to the edge of the glass. If you don't have three to four hours to leave the candle burning the first time you light it then don't do it! Wax has a burn memory, so if you only let it burn halfway to the edge, the candle will continue to melt that far and work its way down into the centre of the wax ('tunnelling'), which will mean your candle won't last nearly as long and you'll be wasting half the wax. You also don't need to trim the wick the first time you burn your candle.

Trimming the wick

Trimming the wick in between each use is essential to ensure that your candle lasts as long as possible and burns evenly and cleanly. A lot of people recommend specialist wick trimmers, but scissors work just as well. Your wick should be around one eighth to one quarter of an inch long before you light it again. You don't want to burn your candle for more than four hours at a time, or the wick will form a carbon deposit at the end (that looks like a mushroom), causing it to emit soot and smoke.

Reusing the glass

If you've spent a significant amount of money buying a premium candle, it seems a shame to throw away the beautiful glass after it's finished. I like to reuse mine for storing makeup brushes and eyeliners, or for desk tidies, which look especially nice using brands like Diptyque and Jo Malone. All you need to do to get a perfectly clean glass is to fill your used candle glass with boiling water right to the top. Stir it for a few seconds to encourage the wax at the bottom to melt, then leave it for a few minutes for it to float to the top. Using a teaspoon or kitchen knife, carefully dislodge the base of the wick. This is usually glued to the bottom of the pot, so the hot water helps to melt the glue and makes it easier to remove. Remove the metal base from the water and leave the water to cool. Once it has cooled, the wax will solidify on the surface of the water. You can then remove it in one piece, empty out the remaining water and pop the glass in the dishwasher on a high heat to remove any tiny bits of residue.

Tip If you're lighting a deep candle and your match or lighter isn't long enough, try lighting the end of a piece of dried spaghetti, then using that as your match!

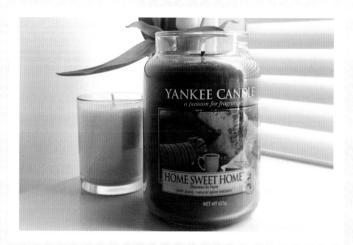

MY FAVOURITE CANDLES

Jo Malone Pomegranate Noir

Jo Malone candles are the ultimate treat and Pomegranate Noir is my favourite home scent of theirs. I had these candles burning at my wedding so the scent will always remind me of that day! It's a warm, rich, yet fruity scent that I usually burn in my living room.

Bath & Body Works Leaves

I pick a few of these candles up whenever I'm in the States during the autumn or winter. It's a seasonal candle so not available in spring and summer, but its warm, spicy fragrance is my all-time favourite. The Bath & Body Works candles kick off so much scent they are great value for money and often on offer. I love burning this candle in my hallway as its scent is so warm and welcoming.

Diptyque Baies

My favourite Diptyque scent and one of their classics, this is a rich cassis and rose fragrance that is homely and fruity at the same time. If you like Pomegranate Noir, you'll love this. It's expensive but makes for a beautiful gift. This is a gorgeous scent for your bedroom or bathroom.

Yankee Candle Home Sweet Home

I've been a fan of Yankee Candles for years and I especially love their Christmas limited-edition scents. My favourite scent of theirs is Home Sweet Home, which is a perfect choice for a kitchen as it's sweet and spicy.

Capri Blue Volcano Candles

You can pick up a wide selection of Capri Blue candles from Anthropologie and they make the same scents in lots of different shapes and colours of jar so it's easy to find one that will go perfectly in your home. My favourite scent is Volcano. It's quite a sweet tropical-citrus fragrance but somehow still warm. It's a perfect scent for a bathroom but works in any room of the house!

Hosting at Home

I love having people to stay. I think it comes from my mum being a natural host and our house always being full of different people from all over the world growing up. My family home has always had that great open door feeling and everyone feels at home there. I always try my best to make any guests feel extra welcome, as staying in someone else's home can be awkward if you feel like they aren't prepared for you (especially for longer periods of time). There are a couple of things I like to do to ensure my guests feel comfortable and at home.

Before they arrive, I always put out a water bottle and glass by the bed, fresh towels and face cloths in the bathroom or on the end of their bed, any toiletries they might need and I always keep a few extra new toothbrushes just in case someone forgets theirs! If you ever stay in a nice hotel and don't need to use the mini toiletries you get in the bathroom they are perfect to take home for the guest room. If you have a spare dressing gown, that's also a nice added touch for your guests.

I like to stock up the spare room with a few magazines and books too, especially if your guests are from overseas and might be suffering from jet lag. There's nothing worse than being awake in the middle of the night in someone else's house with nothing to do! It's also a thoughtful touch to keep a phone charger by the bed just in case, and if you have the time before they arrive, light a scented candle so their room smells divine while they settle in. I also like to turn on the bedside table lights and leave the main lights off for a softly lit, warm feel when they first come into the room. These very small touches make all the difference when you're away from home and will make your guests feel like they are staying in a smart hotel!

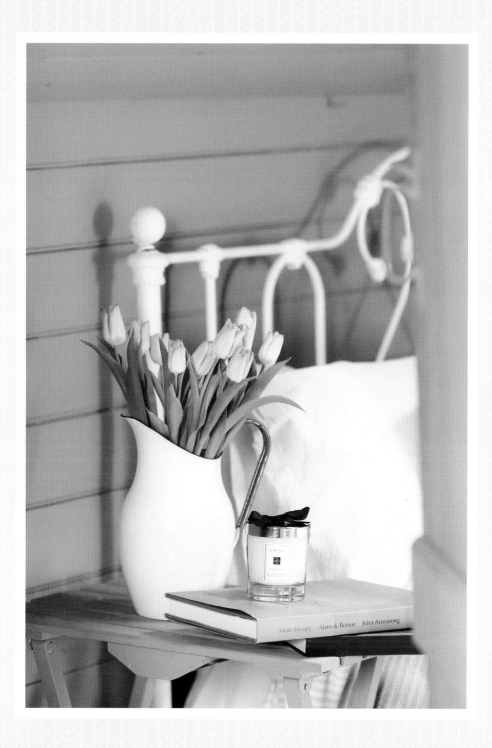

3 Easy Home DIY Projects

You don't have to spend a fortune to refresh the look of your home; there are some really striking, affordable DIY tricks you can use to give your home an instant update, only spending a few pounds. Here are my favourites.

MARBLE AND COPPER BEDSIDE TABLES

Bedside tables can be one of the hardest pieces of furniture to get right, and surprisingly expensive. This simple idea is so quick, easy and it looks a lot more expensive than it is! You can also choose different heights or styles of waste paper bin to make side tables for your living room, or even cluster tables that fit together. The latter works especially well with hexagonal tiles: you can fit them together to make one larger table or separate them for smaller side tables, which also look great if you mix your metals on the base.

You will need
* 2 wire waste paper baskets – the ones in these pictures are from H&M Home, and at time of print they have a great selection, but you can choose any style you like. Ikea also make similar ones that would work well
* Spray paint in a colour of your choice (optional)
* 2 tiles of your choice. These are easy to find in DIY or tile shops – I used leftover tiles from my bathroom floor. You can use any shape or material you like. I prefer white marble (or marble effect) but wood and black marble look both look great too
* A glue gun (optional)

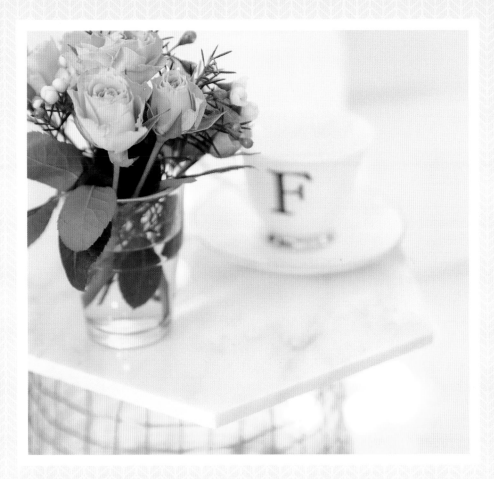

Step 1 Personalise your wire basket. You can use spray paint to spray it a different colour entirely, or even spray half of it for an ombre effect, or leave it as it is if you like the finish already.

Step 2 Wait for it to dry before gluing the base of your basket to the bottom of the tile. This step is optional and just to keep the table-top in place.

If you're using real stone tiles they will be very heavy so don't rely on the glue to hold the tile's entire weight – it's more to stop the top moving around during day-to-day use.

Step 3 Carefully turn your table over and you've got an instant, affordable and stylish little table in about five minutes!

PAINT SWATCH MONTHLY CALENDAR

This little DIY project is perfect for those who like to stay organised, and looks great in an office. You can tailor it to suit your colour scheme and it can stay up year-on-year as it's adjusted using a wipeable marker pen.

You will need

* 35 paint swatches of your choice from a paint book (available for free from your local DIY shop). Try to pick the colours with the biggest swatches, as you'll have more space to write
* A3 or A4 picture frame of your choice – use an A4 one if you want a smaller calendar
* A3 or A4 sheet of wrapping paper or plain coloured paper
* Paper glue – Pritt Stick will do, Spray Mount is even better as it's easier to get a perfect, even finish
* Slim-nibbed marker pen (washable)
* A hole punch or simple round stickers
* A4 printout of the days of the week

Step 1 Decide what colour scheme you want to go for and cut out the appropriate colour swatches from your paint chart. You may need five to seven copies of the same paint chart depending on the pattern your decide to go for, so it's worth working this out when you're in the shop picking them up!

Step 2 Use either a hole punch or simple round stickers in a colour of your choice to make a small circle in the centre at the top of each paint swatch (this will later be used to write the date in).

Step 3 Using a computer, print out the days of the week onto a sheet of paper in a colour of your choice. Cut them out carefully in even, rectangular shapes and cut out one single plain white rectangle from the same sheet of paper (for the title).

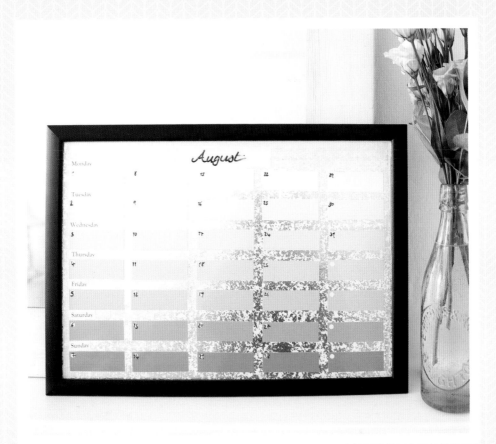

Step 4 Roll out your wrapping paper and glue on your colour swatches in order, running seven across and five down. Then glue on your days of the week above each vertical row and your plain title piece of paper at the top.

Step 5 Frame your paper, then the marker can be used to number the days of the month on the glass over the little round dots. You can then write your appointments on the glass and at the end of the month can be removed easily with a cloth. Write the name of the current month in the space at the top and you're good to go.

HANGING ROPE SHELF

This hanging rope shelf is really simple, but effective and useful at the same time. You can add accent edges using metallic or coloured paint and hang it from the ceiling or wall. You can also make more than one shelf by using extra pieces of wood and knotting them underneath each one. They work really well as bookshelves, in bathrooms for storage and even as bedside tables if you choose a squarer piece of wood.

You will need

* A plank of wood – the shape depends on the type of shelf you want to make, but generally a long rectangle made of an attractive-looking wood like oak works best
* Wood stain or paint in a colour of your choice (this is optional: if you like the colour of your wood plain, skip this)
* A small pot of metallic or coloured paint for the edges of your shelf – also optional but I love to use metallic paint for this as I think it adds a really nice detail
* Thick rope. The length you require depends on how high you want to hang your shelf. Have a think about that before heading to your local DIY shop so you can ensure you have enough
* 2 large metal hooks or loops to hang the rope from the wall or ceiling – make sure these are wide enough to fit your chosen rope through
* A drill – and someone who knows how to use it if you don't!

Step 1 Start by staining or painting your wood if you are going to do so. If you want a whitewashed effect, try watering down plain white wood paint or using a light stain. Wait for it to completely dry, preferably overnight, before moving on.

Step 2 Add your accent paint along the edges of the wood and wait for that to dry.

Step 3 Drill four holes just wide enough for your chosen rope to fit through on each corner of your piece of wood and clean out the holes with a vacuum cleaner to make sure you've got any loose shavings.

Step 4 Drill in appropriate holes to attach your metal hooks or loops to the wall or ceiling.

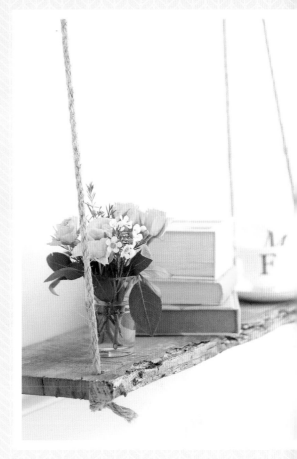

Step 5 Run your rope from underneath the back corner of your wood and knot it on the underside. Run the rope up behind your hook or loop, through it and down again into the front hole on the same side of your wood. Adjust the height accordingly and knot it underneath, cutting off any excess. Repeat for the other side, making sure both sides of the rope are exactly even before tying the final knot tightly!

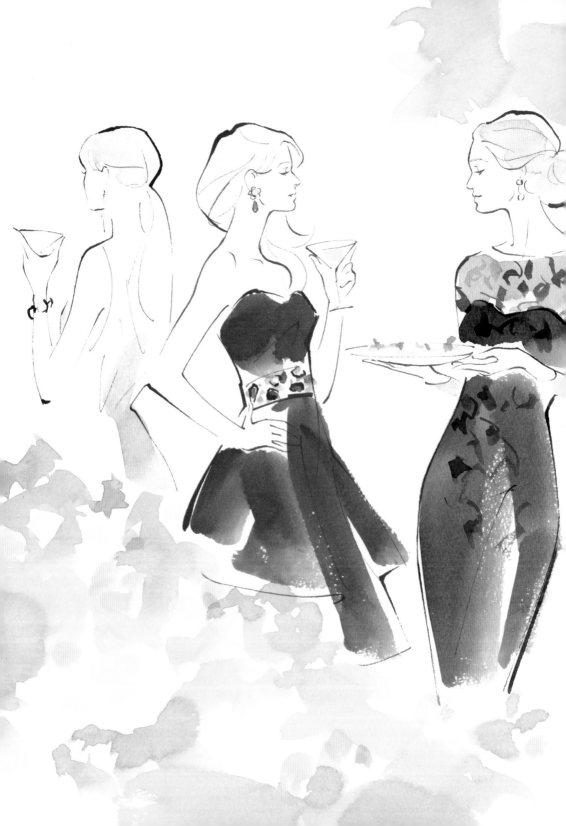

Perfect Party Food

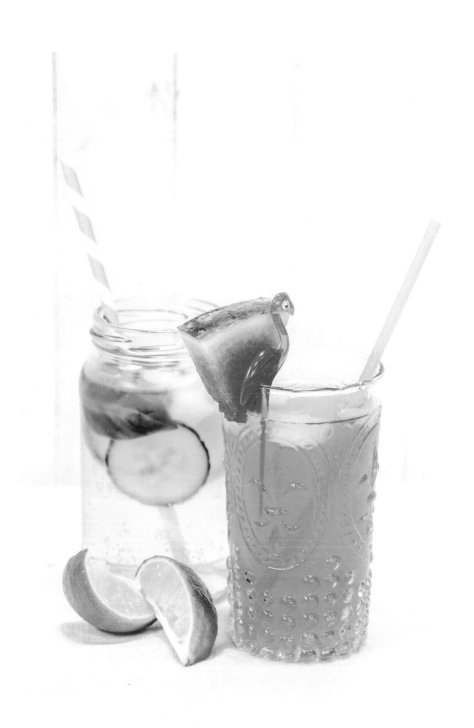

Easy At-Home Cocktails

KILNER JAR GIN AND TONIC

Gin and tonic is my all-time favourite drink and it's really easy to put your own twist on it by replacing a simple slice of lime with something a little different. The following is my personal favourite combination, and it's even better made in a big Kilner jar with a tap so you don't have to keep mixing so many ingredients together. You can get one of these online for around £15 and they're great for summer parties.

25ml gin
25ml elderflower cordial
Juice of ¼ lime

2 slices of cucumber
4 basil leaves
200ml tonic water

WATERMELON APEROL SPRITZ

One of my favourite summer drinks, an Aperol Spritz is the perfect balance of sour yet refreshing. Adding watermelon into the mix makes it even more delicious and perfect for any summer occasion.

25ml Aperol
50ml Prosecco
50ml watermelon juice (to make
    watermelon juice at home, put the
    watermelon flesh into a blender,
    then sieve out any remaining pulp)

Splash of ginger beer
Lots of ice
Slice of watermelon (to garnish)

MOCHA MARTINI

My twist on my favourite pick-me-up cocktail, a mocha martini is slightly sweeter than a traditional espresso martini thanks to the addition of cocoa powder. A perfect date-night drink, or post-dinner treat. Thoroughly mix the cocoa powder into the espresso when it's still hot, then shake all of the ingredients together over ice. You can even garnish it with a few coffee beans for a professional touch.

25ml espresso
1 teaspoon cocoa powder
25ml vodka
25ml Kahlua
1 handful of ice

BERRY SLUSHIE

One of my favourite fruit cocktails, this recipe works especially well in a Nutribullet, but any blender will do the trick. It's so simple to make, you just blend all of the ingredients together and serve. I like to garnish it with a sprig of mint too, and you can also add a leaf or two into the mix for an added touch. If you've got a sweet tooth, add a little more sugar.

25ml white rum
2 handfuls frozen, mixed berries (raspberries,
strawberries and blueberries work best)
1 tablespoon sugar
Juice of ½ lime
1 handful of ice
50ml water
Mint leaves (to garnish)

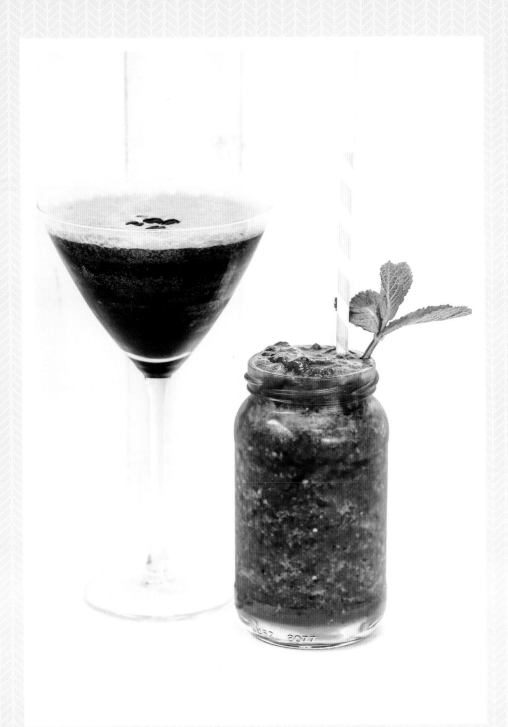

5 Quick Canapé Recipes

CHICORY AND GORGONZOLA BITES

I fell in love with a recipe similar to this when we were filming a cooking series for YouTube a couple of years ago. I've tweaked it to make it even creamier by adding avocado. A lot of similar recipes also include walnuts, but I'm not a huge fan of them personally although you can add them in if you want to.
(Makes approx 20 pieces)

Ingredients
1 ripe avocado
100g Gorgonzola cheese
50g dried cranberries
2 chicories

1. Peel and mash the avocado.
2. Chop the Gorgonzola into small cubes.
3. Roughly mix the avocado, Gorgonzola cubes and dried cranberries together in a bowl.
4. Separate each chicory leaf and place it facing up on a plate (like a spoon).
5. Place a teaspoon of your mixture into each chicory leaf.

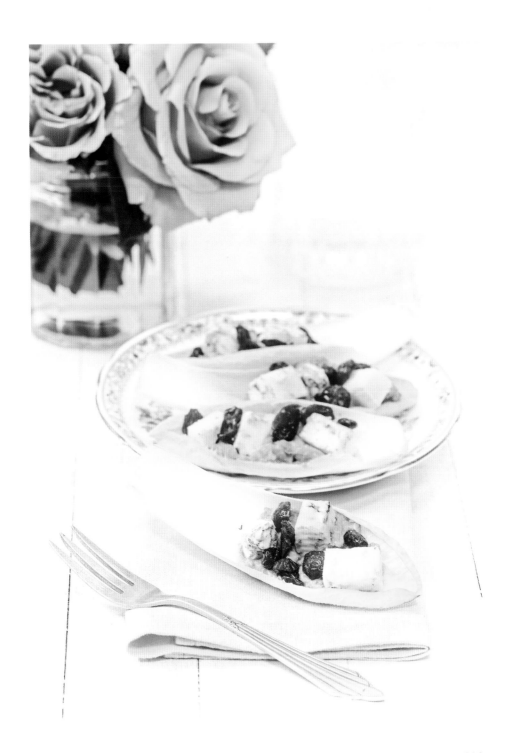

WATERMELON AND FETA SKEWERS

One of the most simple canapés to make, these watermelon and feta skewers feature one of my favourite food combinations (if you like these ingredients together too, watch out for a great salad recipe later in this chapter). You can omit the pancetta for a vegetarian version that's still super tasty.
(Makes approx 18–20 pieces)

Ingredients
¼ medium watermelon
200g Feta cheese
6 slices pancetta

1. Cut the watermelon and Feta into similarly sized cubes.
2. Roughly chop the pancetta slices into thirds.
3. Skewer one piece of each ingredient together on cocktail sticks and season with a tiny bit of black pepper.

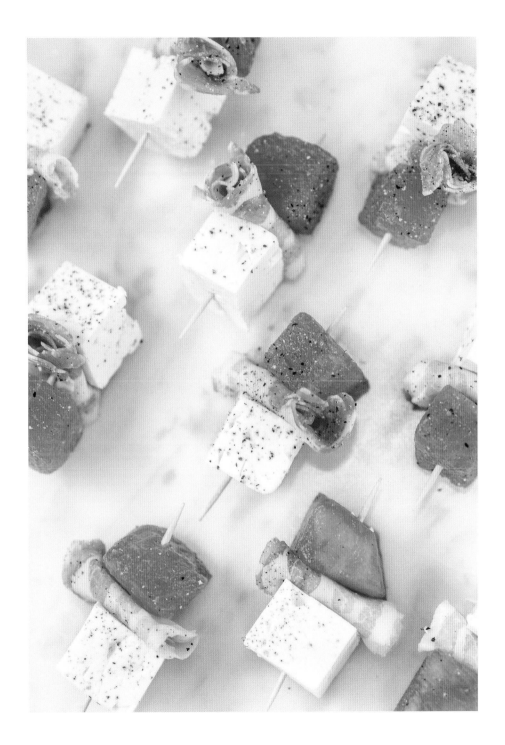

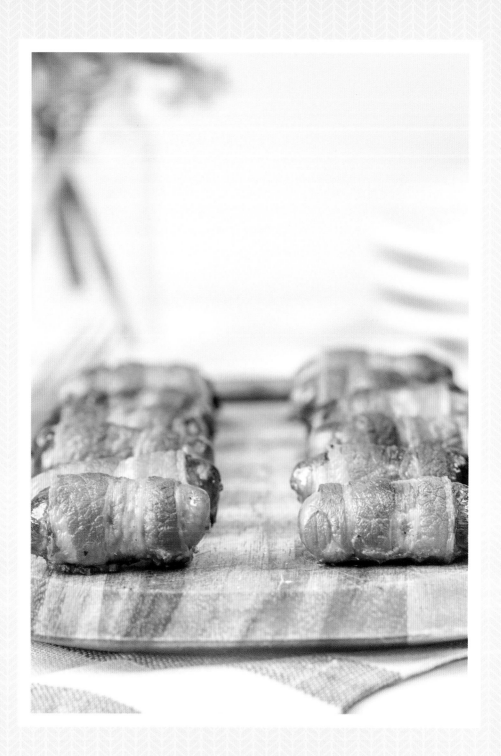

HONEY AND ROSEMARY PIGS IN BLANKETS

My variation on a classic winter treat. Pigs in blankets are a favourite in my family, especially at Christmas, but making your own is a great idea as you can make them a little bit different and they're tastier than the shop-bought alternative.

(Makes approx 24)

Ingredients

12 pork chipolatas
12 bacon rashers
3 sprigs of rosemary
Honey (to glaze)

1. Twist each chipolata into two pieces and cut with scissors to make 24 smaller sausages.
2. Cut each bacon rasher in half, then wrap the sausage in the bacon, crossing over each end.
3. Tuck a little sprig of rosemary underneath the bacon on top of each sausage.
4. Cover the top length of each sausage with a teaspoon of honey and place on a baking tray.
5. Bake in the oven at 190°C/gas mark 5 for 20 minutes.

GNOCCHI BITES

Although traditionally a main dish, gnocchi is perfect for using in canapés as it's bite-sized and works really well when skewered together with a few ingredients. My personal favourite is below, but get creative and make up your own combination of toppings.

(Makes approx 20 pieces)

Ingredients

20 pieces gnocchi
5 sundried tomatoes
20 basil leaves
Drizzle of olive oil

1. Boil the gnocchi for 2–3 minutes until soft, then drain.
2. Chop each sundried tomato into quarters.
3. Make 20 individual skewers using cocktail sticks, each including a piece of the cooked gnocchi, one basil leaf and one quarter of a sundried tomato.
4. Drizzle with olive oil and season with a little salt and pepper before serving.

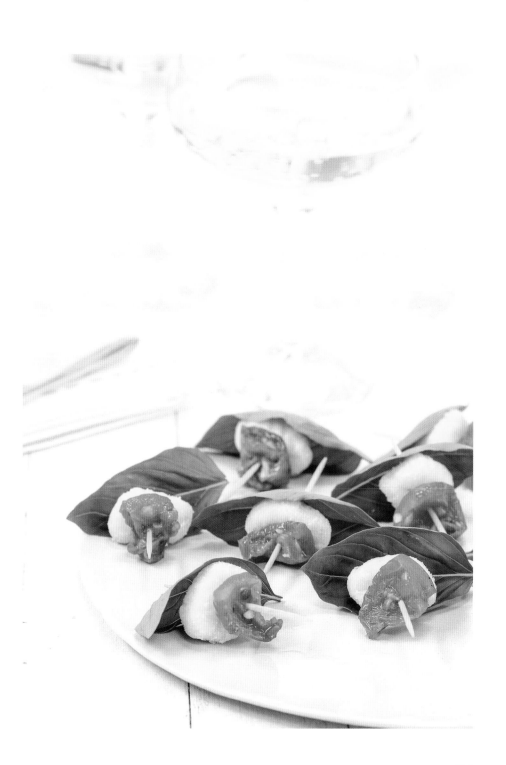

SMOKED SALMON STARS

A little different to your usual smoked salmon and cream cheese canapés, these star-shaped bites are one of my favourite treats for Christmas parties. (Makes approx 20 pieces)

Ingredients
2 large, ripe avocados
Sprinkle of dried chilli flakes
5 slices multi-seed bread
5 slices smoked salmon
10 pitted green olives

You will also need:
medium-sized star-shaped
cookie cutter

1. Peel and mash both avocados until smooth, then season with salt and pepper and mix in a sprinkle of chilli flakes (or more if you like spicy food!).
2. Toast your slices of bread and cut four star shapes out of each one.
3. Divide your smoked salmon slices into quarters and place each on one of your toast stars.
4. Add a heaped teaspoon of your avocado mix into the centre of each star.
5. Slice your olives in half and top off each star with one.

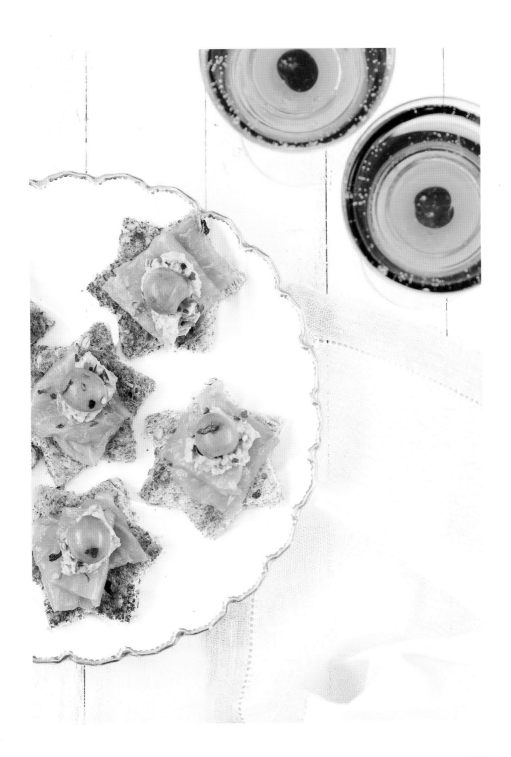

Dinner-Party Staples

COTTAGE PIE

One of the easiest things to throw together if you're feeding a lot of people, cottage pie is equally delicious as a last-minute fix or planned ahead for a chilled-out evening in. I like to spice things up a little bit by adding some chilli but if you don't fancy that, feel free to replace it with some chopped thyme for a more traditional flavour.

(Serves 6)

Ingredients

1.5 kg potatoes, peeled

6 shallots, peeled and
   finely chopped

2 cloves of garlic, crushed

2 tablespoons olive oil

400g lean beef mince
   (I use steak mince from
   a local butcher)

2 carrots, peeled and diced

1 fresh red chilli, chopped

A good splash of red wine

2 tins chopped tomatoes

1 tablespoon gravy granules
   (beef flavour)

150g frozen peas

100g butter

150g mature Cheddar
   cheese, grated

1. Preheat the oven to 180°C/gas mark 4.

2. Cut the potatoes into medium sized chunks, place in a large pan and bring to the boil. Simmer until soft, for around 20 minutes (continue with the rest of the recipe in the meantime!).

3. Throw the shallots and garlic into a thick-bottomed pan with the olive oil and fry for 4 minutes, stirring regularly, so they don't burn but brown evenly.

4. Add the minced beef and carrots and cook until the beef has browned.

5. Add the chilli, red wine and chopped tomatoes. Stir thoroughly and leave to simmer for 15 minutes.

6. Add half your gravy granules. You may find the the mixture thickens sufficiently, but if not, add the other half.

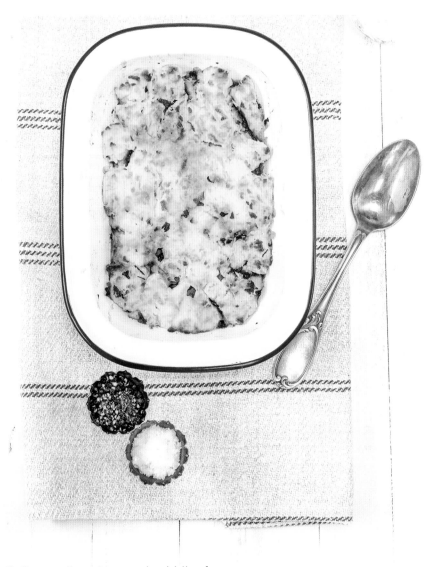

7. Season the mince and add the frozen peas.

8. Drain the potatoes and leave for five minutes. Then mash them adding the butter and seasoning to taste.

9. Pour the mince into a suitably sized oven-proof serving dish. Top with the mashed potato and a generous helping of grated Cheddar.

10. Place in the oven for 30 to 40 minutes until golden and crisping on top.

EASY BEEF WELLINGTON

Beef Wellington is a truly indulgent thing to cook for guests and it's bound to get some majorly positive feedback if you cook it well. It sounds like a scary one, but it's surprisingly easy to make if you take a little extra time to prepare it. It's a great choice if you're feeding 8 to 10 people for a more formal dinner. (Serves 8-10)

Ingredients

1kg beef fillet

Olive oil

Lots of salt
  and cracked
  black pepper

500g puff pastry

250g chestnut
  mushrooms, sliced

Handful of fresh
  tarragon, chopped

180g chicken liver pâté
  or Ardennes pâté

1 tablespoon olive oil

1 egg yolk, beaten

1. Preheat the oven to 220°C/gas mark 7.
2. Oil up the fillet of beef and season it with a generous amount of salt and pepper. Place it on a roasting tray and cook in the oven for approximately 15 minutes (medium rare) or 20 minutes (medium). When it's done put it straight into the fridge to cool for 20 minutes.
3. Reduce the oven temperature to 180°C/gas mark 4.
4. Roll out ⅓ of the puff pastry into a rectangular shape just bigger than your fillet. Place it on a non-stick baking tray. Prick it with a fork and bake for 10–12 minutes.
5. Place the mushrooms and tarragon in a pan with a little oil and fry until all the water that comes out of the mushrooms has evaporated. Leave these to cool.
6. Add the pâté to the mushrooms and mix together.
7. Place the beef fillet on top of the cooked piece of pastry, then cover the top of the beef in the mushroom-pâté mixture.
8. Roll out the remaining puff pastry and cover the beef with it. It needs to be long enough to seal together at the ends, and wide enough to tuck underneath the pre-cooked pastry.

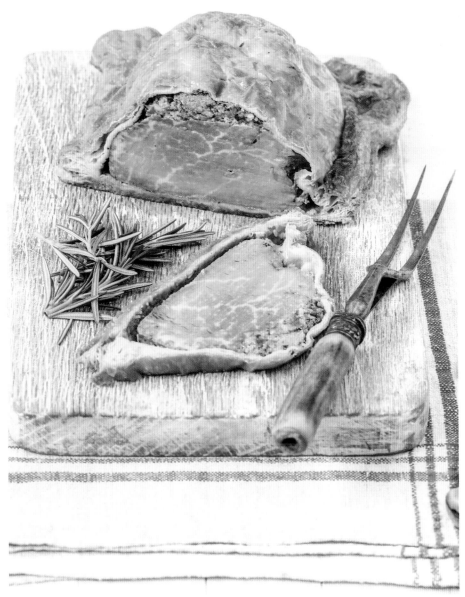

9. Glaze the top with a little beaten egg yolk
10. Return the Wellington to the oven for 15 minutes for medium rare or 25 minutes for medium cooked beef.
11. Remove from the oven and leave for 15 minutes before serving.

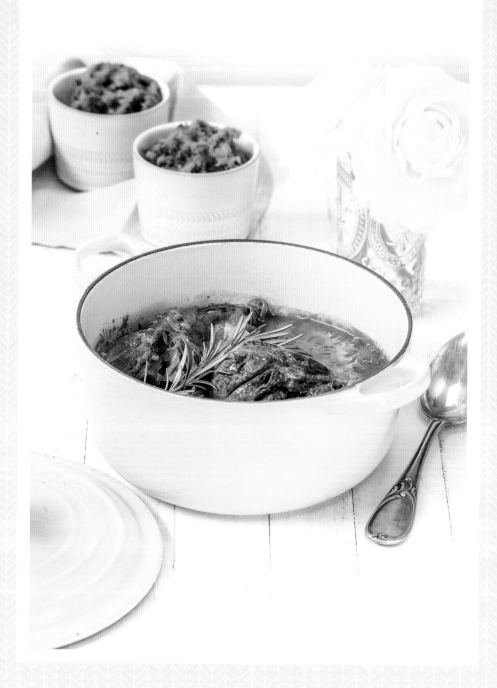

SLOW-COOKED LAMB WITH BUTTERNUT SQUASH MASH

The perfect rich and warming dish to cook for smaller dinner parties. It's really easy to prepare as time does most of the work for you! If you have a slow cooker, you can also make it in that on a low setting over 7–8 hours. (Serves 4)

Ingredients

4 lamb shanks
Olive oil
1 onion, chopped
½ bulb garlic, peeled and chopped
1 glass of red wine
3 sprigs rosemary
2 tins chopped tomatoes
1 lamb stock cube
2 tablespoons balsamic vinegar
2 large butternut squash
1 teaspoon chilli flakes
50g salted butter

1. Preheat the oven to 200°C/gas mark 6.
2. Season the lamb well with salt and pepper, place on a baking tray and roast for 15 minutes to seal. Remove and leave to one side, then turn the oven down to 160°C/gas mark 3.
3. Brown the onions and garlic in a large casserole, then add the wine, rosemary, chopped tomatoes, the stock cube and balsamic vinegar.
4. Finally, add 250ml boiling water and the lamb shanks.
5. Bring back to the boil on the stove then put the lid on and place in the oven for 2 hours.
6. Peel the butternut squash and de-seed. Chop into even pieces about 7cm by 2cm. Spread over a roasting tray, season, drizzle with olive oil and sprinkle on a few chilli flakes. Around 45 minutes before the lamb has finished cooking, turn the oven up to 180°C/gas mark 4 and put the squash in on a low shelf, roasting for around 40 minutes until soft. Remove, then roughly mash the squash with a potato masher, adding the butter.
7. Take out the lamb, check the seasoning and serve with the squash.

HOME-MADE RAVIOLI

Making your own pasta is not only *much* more delicious than buying it from a shop, it's also really fun to do! It's great if you want to do most of the food preparation before your guests arrive, as you can make it earlier in the day and then simply boil it for a few minutes before serving. Alternatively, if you have a small group, it's also quite fun to make together! The recipe below is for ravioli with a sweet potato and goat's cheese filling, but feel free to get creative with the fillings – you can add pretty much anything you like!
(Serves 4)

Ingredients

1kg sweet potatoes, peeled and chopped

120g goat's cheese, crumbled

½ small red chilli, finely chopped and seeds removed

400g pasta flour

3 eggs

Olive oil

1 large handful of rocket per person (to serve)

150g Parmesan cheese (grated, to serve)

1. Roast the sweet potato in a preheated oven at 200°C/gas mark 6 for approximately 25 minutes, then mash until smooth. Add the goat's cheese and chilli, and mix them all together in a bowl. Place to one side.

2. To make the pasta, place 300g of the flour, the eggs and a pinch of salt into a food processor and blend until it forms crumbs.

3. Dust your work surface with some of the remaining flour. Remove the dough from the food processor and knead it together for about 5 minutes until it's smooth.

4. Roll the dough into a ball, wrap it in cling film and put it in the fridge for at least 30 minutes.

5. Re-dust your work surface with flour, then divide the dough into quarters and roll the first quarter out using a large rolling pin. If you have a pasta maker, then now is the time to set it out! Start on the widest setting, rolling it through twice on each setting before moving it down to the next. I stop on the second or third thinnest setting, but if you like really fine pasta, go as thin as you can. Don't forget

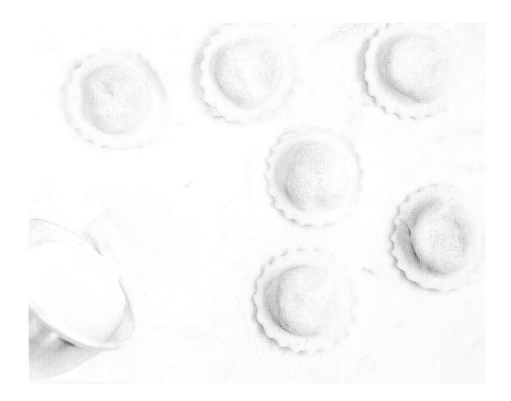

to keep dusting your pasta with flour as you go. If you don't have a pasta machine, you can use your rolling pin to make the pasta as thin as possible. Do the same for the remaining three sections of dough.

6. Use a cookie cutter to cut out as many rounds as you can, then combine all the spare pasta dough and roll through the machine again to get the most pieces from it.

7. Moving quickly once the pasta's rolled (it dries fast!), spoon a teaspoon's worth of filling into the centre of half the pasta shapes, then place another empty pasta shape on top, sealing it with water around the edges and using your fingertips to make sure there are no air bubbles.

8. Leave the ravioli for a few minutes to dry out before cooking it for 4 minutes in a large pan. Make sure you keep the water simmering gently rather than fully boiling, as the ravioli may split.

9. Drain the pasta and serve with a drizzle of olive oil, season with salt and pepper, and garnish with some rocket and grated Parmesan cheese.

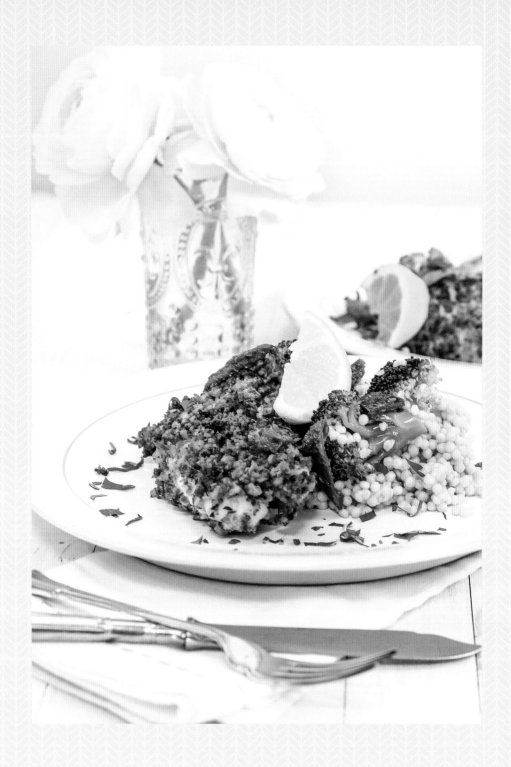

Lighter Entertainment

Healthier Recipes for Hosting at Home

CRISPY BAKED COD WITH GIANT COUSCOUS

This is a great alternative to fried fish and chips as it's much healthier, equally as tasty and the giant couscous means it's also as filling. If you're wondering why to pre-toast the breadcrumbs, it's because then you don't have to overcook your cod to make sure the breadcrumbs are crispy, so make sure you don't leave this step out! This way you get perfectly cooked fish with a super-crispy crust.

(Serves 4)

Ingredients

4 pieces sliced white
    bread or 220g pre-made
    breadcrumbs
1 clove garlic, crushed
Handful of chopped mixed
    herbs; try flat-leafed parsley,
    basil and chives
Zest of 1 lemon
Olive oil

1 egg yolk
4 x 150g cod fillets
    (thick fillets work best)
½ fish stock cube
150g giant couscous
150g broccoli, cut into
    small florets
6 sundried tomatoes

1. Preheat the oven to 180°C/gas mark 4.
2. Cut the crusts off the bread, then whizz it in a food processor to make breadcrumbs (if you don't have a food processor, use pre-made breadcrumbs).
3. Add the garlic, parsley, basil, chives and lemon zest, then stir to combine.
4. Place the breadcrumb mixture in a frying pan with a dash of olive oil and toast gently until it starts to brown, then remove from the heat.
5. Whisk up the egg yolk and coat each cod fillet with egg, then press on the breadcrumbs until the fish is evenly covered.
6. Place the fillets onto a wire rack on top of a baking tray and bake them in the oven for approximately 8-12 minutes.
7. In the meantime, bring a pan of water to the boil, dissolve ½ a fish stock cube and add the couscous. Boil for 8 minutes before adding the broccoli, then boil for a further 5 minutes before draining and returning to the pan.
8. Cut the sundried tomatoes into quarters and add them to the pan. Mix together and serve with the cod fillets.

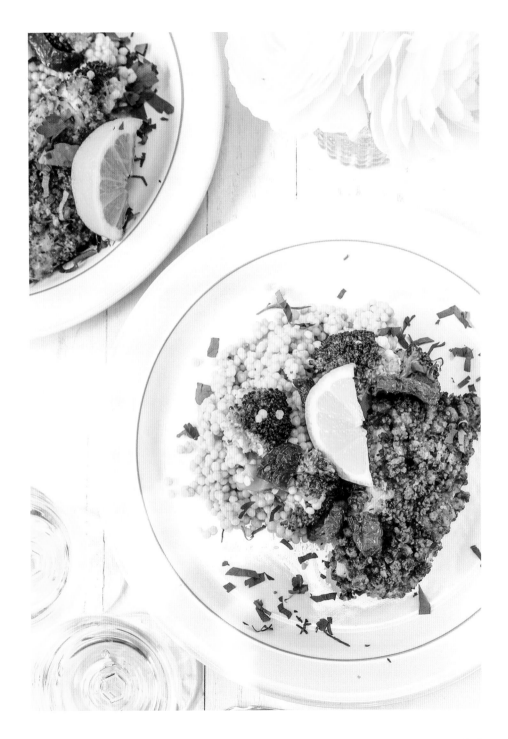

QUINOA WITH CHICKEN AND GOAT'S CHEESE

Quinoa is one of my favourite comfort-food replacements when I want to go for a more healthy option as it has a really comforting texture. I actually prefer mine on the well-cooked side as it's slightly softer and sticks together, a little like mashed potato. This recipe is one I often cook at home for myself or when I'm entertaining, as it's really simple but exceptionally tasty and healthy to boot. It works equally well on its own for a simple dinner, or as an accompaniment to meat or fish if you remove the chicken from the recipe.

(Serves 4 as a main or 8 as a side)

Ingredients

2 cloves garlic, crushed

1 small onion, finely sliced

Olive oil (or avocado oil if you prefer)

3 x 200g chicken breast fillets, diced

100g chestnut mushrooms, sliced

Handful of fresh tarragon, chopped

250g precooked white and red quinoa

100g goat's cheese, crumbled

Generous amount of chopped parsley

1. Put the garlic and onions into a large frying pan with a good slug of olive oil. Fry gently for 3-4 minutes.
2. Add the chicken and cook for a further 3 minutes.
3. Then add the mushrooms and tarragon. Cook for a further 8 minutes or so until the chicken is cooked through.
4. Add the quinoa to the pan and stir well. Cook for another 2–3 minutes before crumbling in the goat's cheese and seasoning the mixture to taste. Stir again to make sure the ingredients are fully combined, then remove from the heat and serve with a generous amount of chopped parsley.

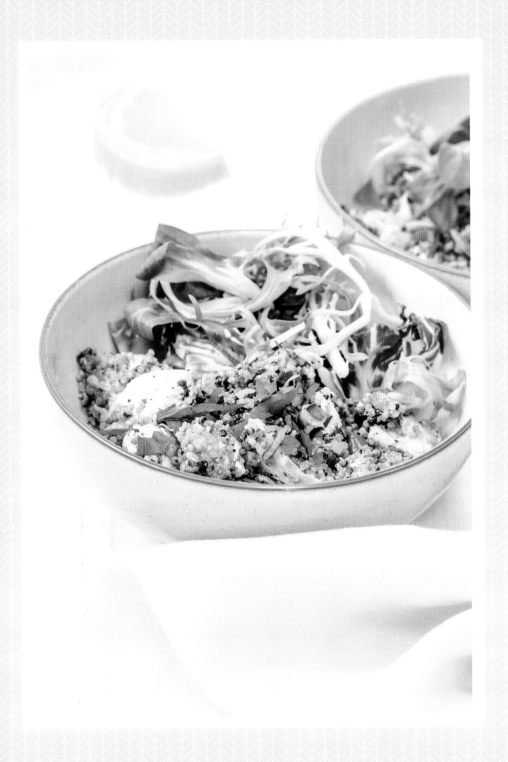

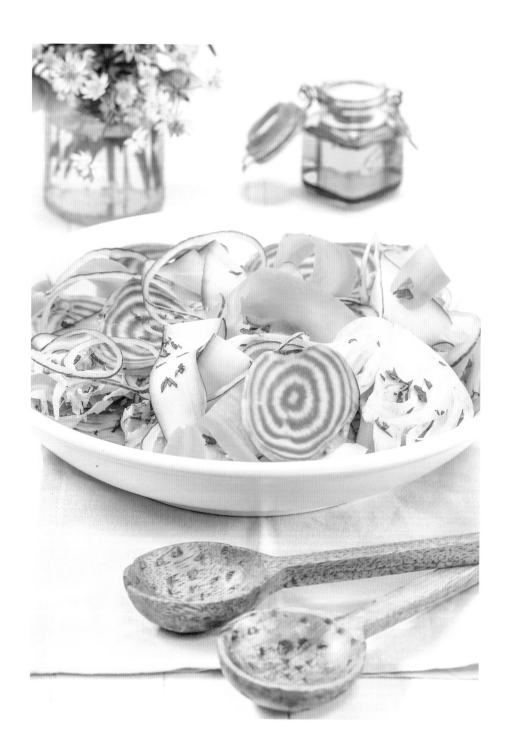

SHAVED RAW VEGETABLE SALAD

This colourful raw vegetable salad recipe is so simple to make and tastes amazing. It's a perfect lunch recipe for big groups but would also work really well as a side at a dinner party. The bright colours mean it looks vibrant on a plate and works especially well in the summertime. I would really recommend investing in a mandolin if you want to try this recipe out, as it's the thinness of the slices that make this salad special.

(Serves 4)

Ingredients
½ cabbage
1 courgette
1 large beetroot
1 fennel
2 carrots
1 red onion
50ml olive oil
50ml balsamic vinegar
6–8 sprigs of fresh mint
100g Gorgonzola cheese

1. Using a mandolin, slice all of the vegetables into super-thin slices and combine in a bowl. (Be very careful – mandolins are sharp! If you're inexperienced using one, it's a good idea to wear rubber gloves.).
2. In a jar, combine the olive oil and the balsamic vinegar.
3. Finely chop 10 mint leaves and pop these into the jar, replace the lid and shake well to make the dressing. Pour the dressing over the vegetables and thoroughly mix everything together.
4. Divide the salad onto four plates.
5. Chop the Gorgonzola into small cubes and divide between the four plates, scattering the cubes on top of the salad.
6. Garnish each with a sprig of mint.

LENTIL LASAGNE

This vegetarian lasagne is a great choice when you're cooking for a bigger group that consists of both veggies and meat eaters, as it's not only healthy and delicious but it's also really filling. It's exceptionally easy to make vegan with the addition of soy milk and egg-free pasta sheets too, which you can pick up from larger supermarkets.

(Serves 4-6)

Ingredients

1 large onion, finely chopped

2 cloves garlic, crushed

150g leeks, sliced

100g mushrooms, sliced

1 teaspoon dried oregano

1 vegetable stock cube

Olive oil

1 tin chopped tomatoes

250g pre-cooked Puy lentils

2 heads cauliflower, cut into small florets

60ml milk

150g grated Parmesan cheese (but not for the vegan version!)

8-10 sheets of lasagne pasta

1. Preheat the oven to 180°C/gas mark 4.
2. Chuck the onion, garlic, leeks, mushrooms, oregano and the stock cube into a pan with a generous amount of olive oil and gently cook until soft for 8 minutes.
3. Add the chopped tomatoes, a can full of water and the lentils. Stir together and season, then leave to simmer for 15 minutes. This sauce will get thick and stodgy, which is perfect.
4. Boil the cauliflower until just soft - around 5 to 6 minutes - then drain and leave to dry off. Whizz in a food processor with the milk until smooth. Season this well with salt and lots of pepper. Then stir in half the Parmesan.
5. In a medium-sized oven dish, layer 1/3 of the lentil mix and 1/3 of the cauliflower mix then cover with sheets of lasagne. Repeat the process with another third of the mixtures. Then for the final layers, put a layer of lasagne between the lentils and the cauliflower.
6. Cover the top with the rest of the Parmesan cheese and bake for 45 minutes.

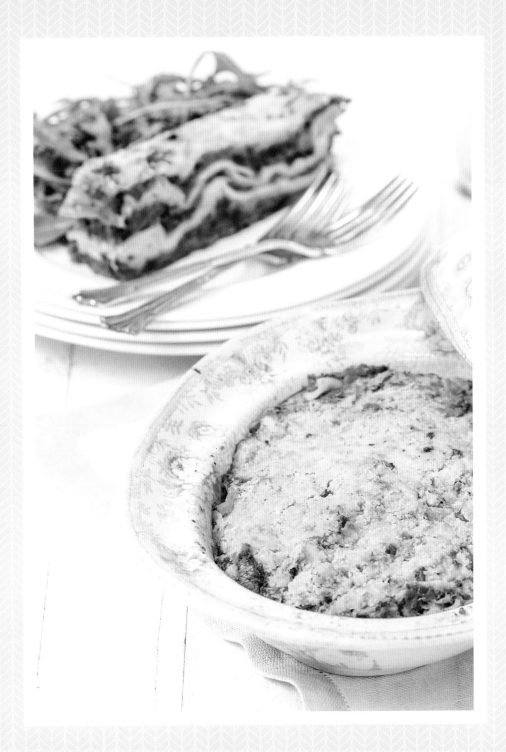

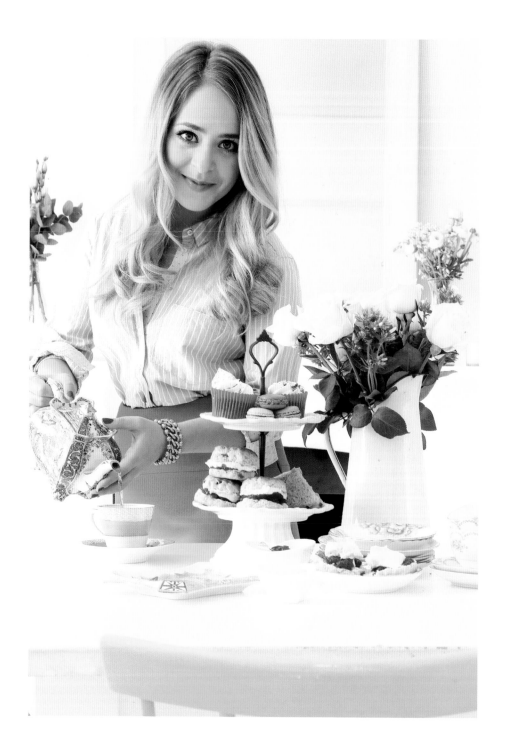

Afternoon Tea Made Easy

Afternoon tea is one of my absolute favourite things to do with my friends at the weekends. It can seem a little daunting to host at home due to the vast selection of food that you usually get, but it doesn't have to be hard work. Here are my top five tips for hosting the perfect afternoon tea without breaking the bank or spending more than a few hours preparing.

Good china doesn't have to cost the earth

Mismatched tea cups look cooler than a matching set anyway, so it's not only cheaper to pick up single teacups at vintage markets and antique auctions but it's also loads of fun! I love browsing antiques with my mum as she's got a great eye for special pieces. You also want to look out for a big teapot – the bigger the better when it comes to afternoon tea as you don't want to be re-filling it all the time. Also keep an eye out for cute tea plates: they sometimes come with the teacup and saucer or can be found alone for just a few pounds.

Simplify your sandwiches

Stick to simple fillings for your sandwiches and it will take you much less time to prepare. My personal favourites are cucumber (a classic afternoon tea sandwich – it's got to be done, with a generous layer of butter!), cheddar and tomato or smoked salmon and cream cheese. All require no cooking or mixing of ingredients. Simple, quick and delicious.

Home-made scones are best

They are a key component to traditional afternoon tea and one of my personal favourites, but they are also really quick and easy to whip up at home! Here's my mum's recipe.

(Makes 12 large scones or 24 mini ones)

Ingredients

250g self-raising flour
50g butter
25g caster sugar
1 teaspoon baking powder
100ml whole milk

1. Preheat the oven to 220°C/gas mark 7.
2. Throw all the ingredients in the food processor except the milk and combine until it forms a breadcrumb texture. Then add your milk a little bit at a time and continue to blend until the mixture forms a ball of dough.
3. Dust your work surface with flour and flatten the dough with your hands (you can use a rolling pin but you don't need to) until it's around 2 cm thick. Then use a cookie cutter to cut out your individual scones.
4. Place on a baking tray and brush the tops with milk, then cook for 10–15 minutes or until they are golden – the time depends on the size of your scone.

You can add in dried fruit or crystallised ginger if you like, but I prefer mine plain (and they are always better if you can serve them warm). When it comes to the cream, always go for clotted cream instead of whipped, as it's less work for you and it tastes amazing. If you want to make your own jam, do so well in advance and keep it in the fridge until you want to use it (if you make a big batch it's also a great gift to give a jar to your friends when they leave). If you do have lots of time on your hands, definitely have a crack at the more complex sweet treats like macarons and éclairs, but if you want to make it easy for yourself, you can always buy the more complex bits. If you mix them in with home-made goodies, I'm sure no one will even notice!

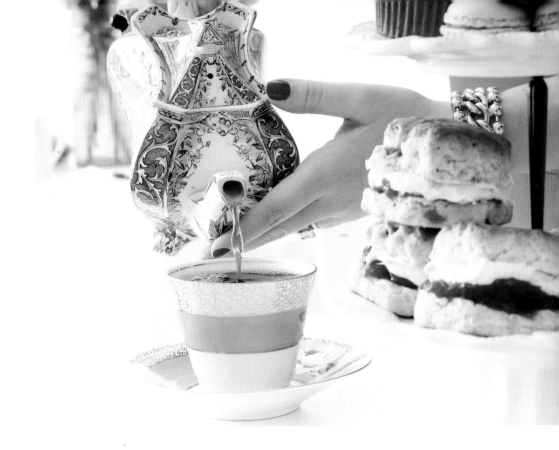

Get creative with your shapes!

Making your tea-time treats in cute shapes will give them the wow factor without having to spend too much extra time actually making them. Scones work especially well when cut into heart shapes instead of rounds (the only change you need to make is the shape of your cookie cutter) and you can even use flower shapes, stars or hearts to cut out your sandwiches instead of the usual rectangles!

Think about your presentation

Traditional cake stands look beautiful, but if you don't have one you can just get creative with whatever's in your kitchen. Wooden chopping boards or slate place mats are perfect to display cakes on, and you can place smaller items in Kilner jars or in teacups themselves (putting your jam and cream in teacups looks cute too). I also like to decorate the table with flowers picked from the garden, simply tied together with a ribbon and popped in a large jam jar.

Martini Glass Puddings

(for the Perfect Portion!)

If you are entertaining for a lot of people, the following three recipes are a great idea if you want to prep ahead of time and have your dessert chilled and ready to serve, already divided into perfect portions. They also look really professional and you can get creative with the presentation too. If you don't have martini glasses at home these also work in wine glasses, tumblers and even shot glasses for mini portions!

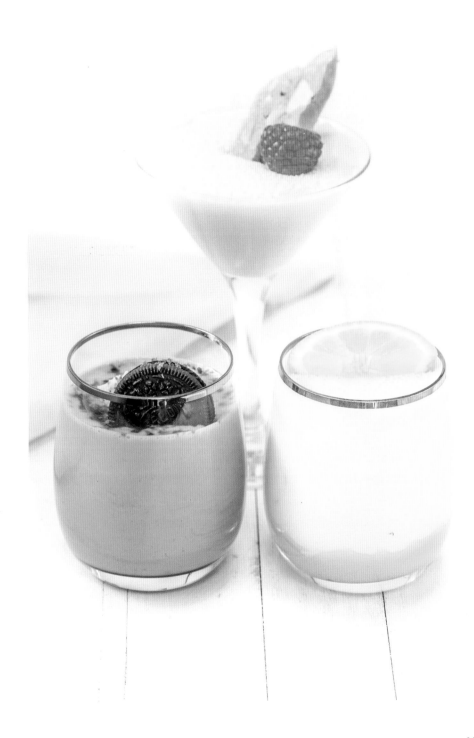

PEANUT BLONDIE MOUSSE

I've never been a huge fan of brownies (call me crazy!) but I adore blondies. This little recipe is super-rich and indulgent, so it's perfect for serving in small portions like this. (Serves 6)

Allergy advice: For allegens (including cereals containing gluten) see asterisked ingredients.

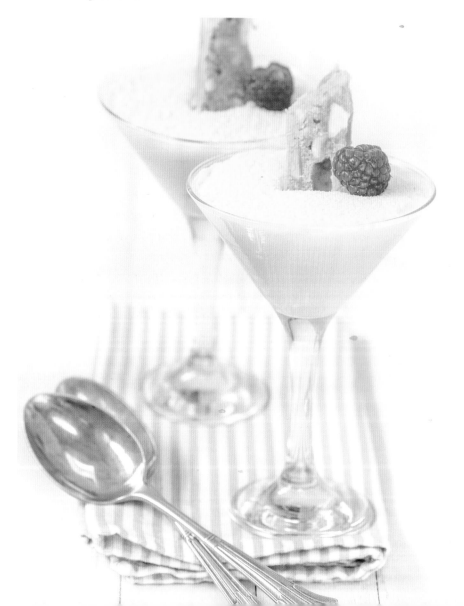

For the blondies:

Ingredients

80g butter

85g light brown sugar

1 egg, beaten

1 teaspoon vanilla
  extract

80g white chocolate
  chips

40g peanuts, roughly
  chopped *

110g plain flour

½ teaspoon baking
  powder

1. Preheat the oven to 160°C/gas mark 3.
2. Melt the butter in a pan over a low heat then pour it into a mixing bowl and set aside.
3. Once the butter has cooled for a couple of minutes, stir in the sugar, egg and vanilla extract until combined, then add the chocolate chips and chopped peanuts.
4. Sieve the flour and baking powder and add to the mixture, combining well so it's smooth and consistent.
5. Pour your mixture into a small baking tray (it doesn't matter too much if you don't have one small enough, just stick to one end and smooth out the mixture till it's about an inch thick). Bake for about 15 minutes before removing. Leave to cool completely then cut into squares.

For the mousse:

Ingredients

250g white chocolate

60ml whole milk

225ml double cream,
  whipped

2 egg whites

Dash of lemon juice

1. Melt the chocolate carefully either in the microwave or in a bowl on top of a pan of simmering water. Then add the milk and combine slowly. Leave this to cool for a good 15 minutes.
2. Slowly stir the whipped-cream in to the chocolate.
3. In a separate bowl, whisk the egg whites with a dash of lemon juice until they form stiff peaks.
4. Carefully fold in the egg whites to the chocolate and cream.
5. Pour into six martini glasses and refrigerate for a minimum of 4 hours. Then take a square of your blondie and slide it into the mousse. Enjoy!

As this recipe contains raw egg whites, do not serve to the elderly, pregnant women, babies and toddlers, or people who are already unwell because of the risk of food poisoning.

LEMON CURD PANNA COTTA

Panna cotta is one of my favourite indulgent treats. This one combines the subtle creaminess of the panna cotta layer with the sharp, tart flavour of another of my favourite treats ... lemon curd!
(Serves 6)

Ingredients

5 sheets of Costa
    Fine Leaf Gelatine
600ml double cream
150ml whole milk
100g caster sugar
2 unwaxed lemons,
    zested and juiced
150g lemon curd
Raspberries
    (to garnish)

1. Slide the leaf gelatine into some cold water for 4 minutes until soft.
2. Put the cream, milk and sugar into a non-stick pan and heat gently until hot, but not boiling. Then stir in the lemon juice and zest and leave to stand for 3 minutes.
3. Remove the gelatine from the cold water, squeeze off any excess and add it to the pan. Stir in until dissolved. Leave the mixture to cool for about 15 minutes.
4. In the meantime, divide the lemon curd between your 6 glasses, making an even layer in each. When the cream mixture is still slightly warm, divide it between the 6 glasses and place it immediately into the fridge.
5. Leave it overnight to set and serve straight from the fridge, with a few raspberries on top for decoration.

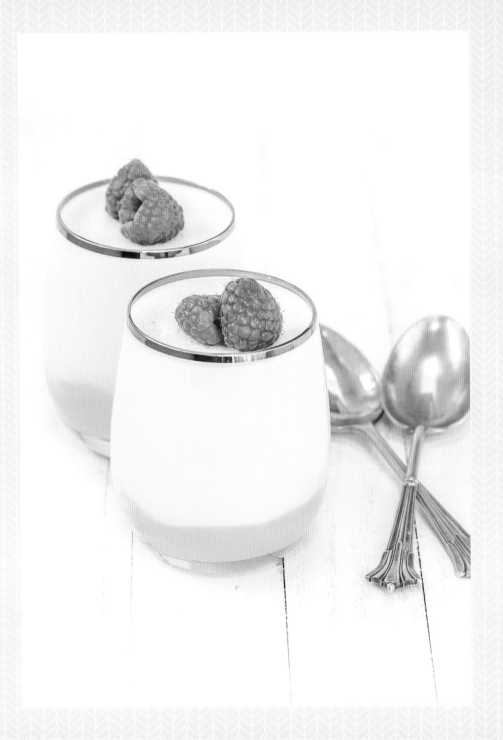

SALTED CARAMEL CREAM PUDDING WITH COOKIES

I absolutely adore the addition of salted caramel to any recipe, but this is perhaps the most delicious one I've ever tried!

(Serves 6)

Ingredients

100g dark brown
  sugar
100ml water
520ml milk
3 tablespoons
  cornflour
5 egg yolks
1½ teaspoons vanilla
  extract
¾ teaspoon flaked
  sea salt
40g butter
6 Oreo cookies
Whipped cream
  (to serve)

1. Heat the sugar and water in a pan over a medium heat until it melts and starts to caramelise. It's useful to have a sugar thermometer for this, as you can be more precise – remove from the heat when it reaches 100°C.

2. Take a separate pan and pour in 60ml milk. Whisk in the cornflour until completely dissolved, then add the rest of your milk. Place your pan on a medium heat and bring almost to a simmer then remove from the heat.

3. Place the egg yolks into a mixing bowl and whisk them together. Then slowly add the milk and cornflour mixture, whisking constantly.

4. Add the cooling caramel, vanilla extract and butter. Then return to the caramel pan. Reheat until very hot but not boiling – about 80°C.

5. Pour into 6 glasses then cover in cling film and put them in the fridge overnight.

6. To serve, place a single Oreo cookie flat on the surface of each serving, with a dollop of whipped cream on top for decoration.

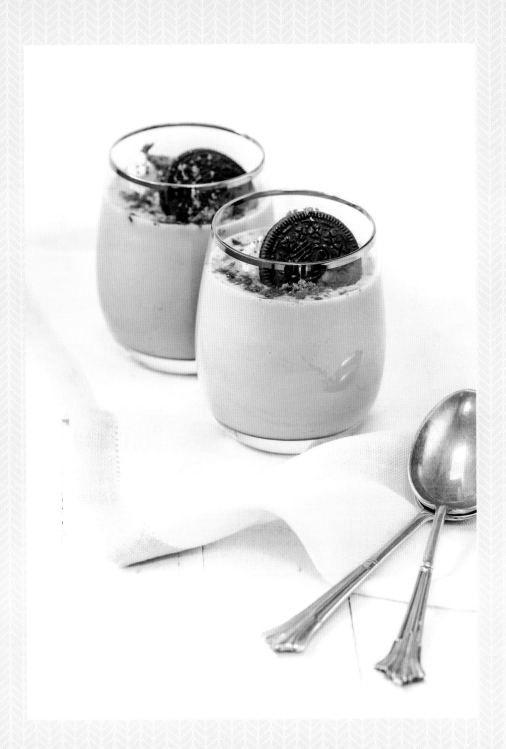

RAINBOW SPRINKLES CUPCAKES

This cupcake recipe is as simple as it gets and pretty enough to impress both children and adults alike. You can make buttercream icing if you intend to keep the cakes for a few days before they are consumed (it lasts longer) but I prefer them served fresh with whipped-cream icing, as below.

(Makes 12 cupcakes)

For the cupcakes:

Ingredients

110g butter

65g sugar

2 eggs

1 tablespoon vanilla extract

190g plain flour

1 teaspoon baking powder

80ml milk

5 tablespoons multi-coloured sprinkles

For the icing:

Ingredients

300ml whipping cream

70g icing sugar

1 teaspoon vanilla extract

Assorted food colourings, as desired

1. Preheat the oven to 180°C/gas mark 4.
2. Mix the butter and sugar together in a food processor until combined (you can do this by hand, but make sure your butter is very soft).
3. Add the eggs and vanilla extract and combine.
4. Sift in your flour and baking powder then gradually add the milk as you mix it.
5. Add your sprinkles and fold them in by hand, then spoon your mixture into cupcake cakes (about two thirds full). Bake for 14 minutes, then remove and cool on a wire rack before icing.
6. For the icing, whisk the cream until it becomes frothy before sifting in the sugar and adding the vanilla extract.
7. Divide the icing into separate bowls according to the number of colours you're using, and add a touch of food colouring to each one (my suggestions would be red, blue and yellow).
8. Continue whisking each until the icing is thick enough to pipe or spread.
9. When your cupcakes are completely cooled, spread icing onto each one using a flat spatula, or pipe it on using a piping bag or freezer bag with the corner cut off.
10. Top off each cake with some more sprinkles and serve as soon as possible.

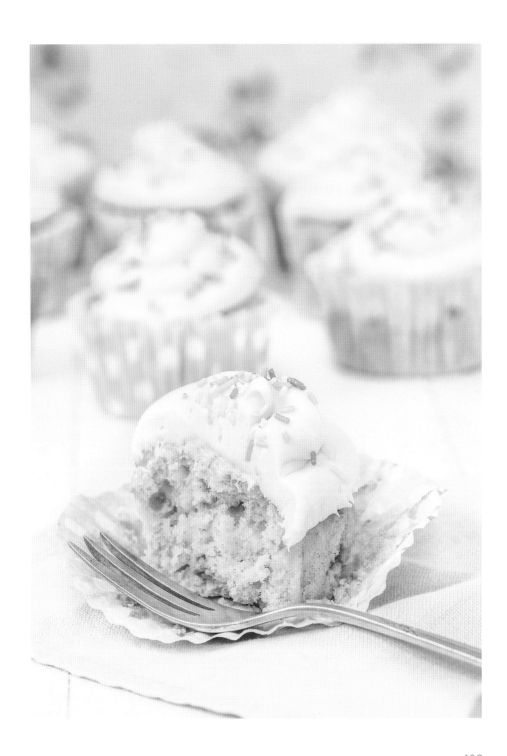

NAKED STRAWBERRIES AND CREAM CAKE

This type of cake has become so popular for weddings over the past few years but it's actually really simple to make. It's more delicious than traditional iced cakes and it also looks beautiful so is the perfect choice for a special occasion.

(Makes 1 large cake that serves approx 20, depending on your portions!)

For the cake mixture:

Ingredients

8 eggs
450g caster sugar
450g self-raising flour
450g butter
4 teaspoons baking powder
2 teaspoons vanilla extract

For the filling:

Ingredients

500ml whipping cream
500g strawberries
1 jar of strawberry jam
Icing sugar for dusting

1. Preheat the oven to 180°C/gas mark 4.
2. Grease and line 4 x 20 cm round cake tins by taking the wrapper from a stick of butter and wiping it around the side of your tin. Cut out a circle of baking paper for the bottom of each tin and place them in there. (If you don't have four tins, you can cook the mixture in batches.)
3. Mix together the eggs, sugar, flour, butter, baking powder and vanilla extract until well combined (either in a food processor or by hand).
4. Divide your mixture into four and separate evenly between the tins, smoothing the surface of each before placing in the oven for 20–25 minutes.
5. Remove from the oven and leave the cakes for 5 minutes to cool before removing them from the tins and placing on a wire rack to cool completely.
6. To make the filling, whip the cream in a large bowl.
7. Slice the strawberries into thin slices.
8. To assemble, place one cake upside down as the base. Spread a layer of jam, followed by a layer of whipped cream, followed by a layer of sliced strawberries, and repeat this with the three other cakes until you have a tall, four-layered cake.
9. Cover the top with a final layer of whipped cream, use sliced or whole strawberries to decorate then sift the whole cake with icing sugar.

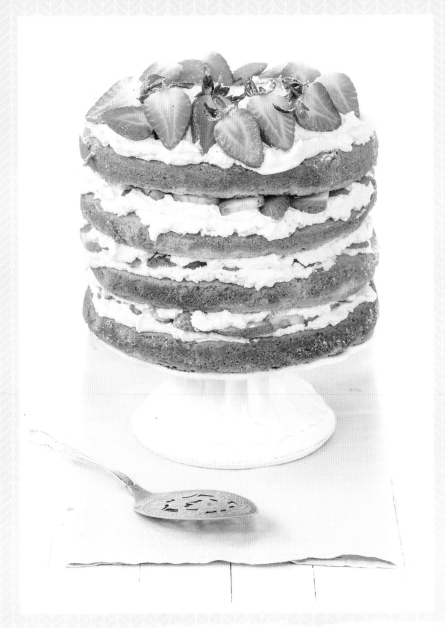

Tip If your cakes rise unevenly (i.e. the middle is much higher than the edge) you can slice off the peaks to make them easier to layer and more stable as a result.

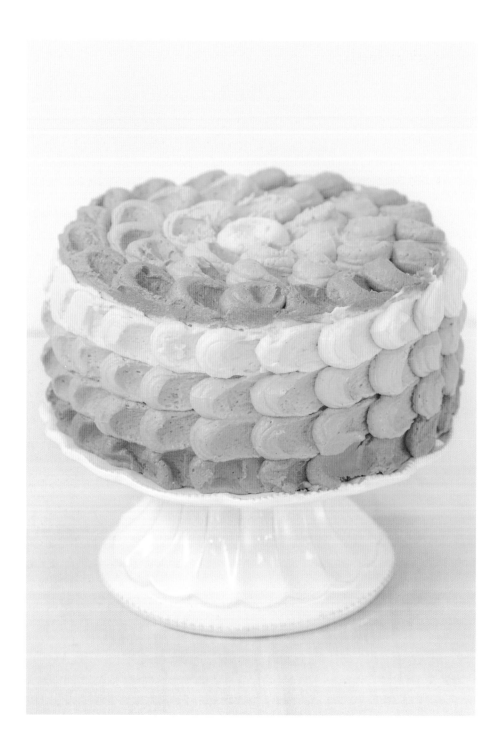

CHOCOLATE OMBRÉ PETAL CAKE

This cake isn't the most simple to assemble, but it's really eye-catching and bound to get an influx of compliments if you pull it off! You can choose what colour to decorate it based on the occasion, or use a rainbow of colours for the most dramatic effect. The cake itself is very simple but you'll need to take a little extra time when it comes to the icing. (Serves 8)

For the cake mixture:

Ingredients

3 eggs
175g self-raising flour
175g caster sugar
175g butter
1 teaspoon of
  baking powder
40g cocoa powder

For the icing:

Ingredients

225g unsalted butter
3 tablespoons
  cream cheese
200g vegetable
  shortening
675g icing sugar
2 tablespoons
  vanilla extract
60ml milk
Food colouring (of
  your choice)

1. Preheat the oven to 180°C/gas mark 4.
2. Beat the eggs, flour, sugar, butter and baking powder until smooth to form a cake batter.
3. In a separate bowl, mix together the cocoa powder with around 4 tablespoons of water until it forms a paste, then add it to the cake batter.
4. Pour the mixture into a small, deep cake tin (the taller your cake is, the more layers of icing will fit onto the sides and the more striking it will look) and bake for 20–25 minutes. Leave to cool in the tin before removing and leaving to cool completely on a wire rack before icing.
5. For the icing, mix together the butter, cream cheese and shortening in a food mixer till smooth. Continue mixing while adding the icing sugar slowly.
6. Next mix in the vanilla extract and a pinch of salt.
7. Keeping the mixer on, start to mix in the milk until you have reached the right consistency for butter cream. Then leave the mixer running for a couple of minutes to ensure everything is fully combined.
8. Divide your icing into 4–6 smaller bowls (depending on the height of your cake!). Leave one bowl white, then add a tiny amount of food colouring into the first bowl, and mix it in. A little bit more into the next bowl, and so on, until you have a nice gradient of colours between the bowls.

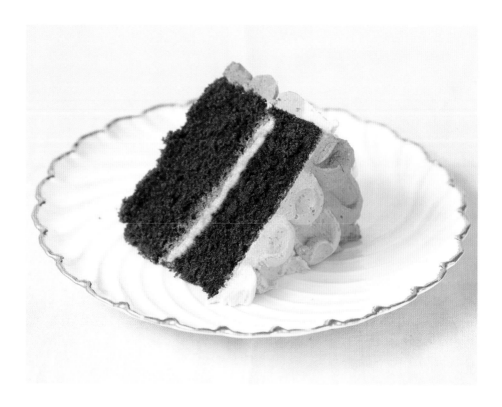

9. Using the same number of piping bags (if you don't have piping bags, you can use freezer bags with the corners cut off), fill each with one colour of your icing. Then put a single dollop of each from the bottom of the cake to the top, starting with the darkest colour, ending up with the lightest. If you have an especially tall cake, or fewer shades of the icing, you can ice two dollops of each, or make each iced dollop larger.

10. Using a small spatula, or the back of a teaspoon, drag one side of each dollop outwards (sideways across the side of the cake).

11. Then place the next line of icing just before the end of the 'tail' of each icing dollop, and repeat.

12. When you get all the way around the cake, finish off the final gap with a single row of icing and don't spread it out using the spatula (this can be the back of the cake!).

13. For the top, you can decorate it any way you want with the remainder of the icing.

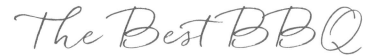
The Best BBQ

My Favourite Outdoor Dishes and Summer Specialities

AT-HOME BBQ MARINADE

Once you perfect a great BBQ marinade at home, it can work as the basis
for loads of your barbecue recipes, from ribs to chicken, steak and veggies.
It's really simple to make so there's no point in splashing out for pre-made
marinades that can be expensive and processed. Here's my favourite recipe,
which you can (and should) tweak to your own tastes, adding spices and herbs
as you like – get creative!

Ingredients

4 cloves garlic

1 large onion

1 small fresh red chilli

3 tablespoons
   brown sugar

1 teaspoon English
   mustard

1 tablespoon olive oil

100ml ketchup

30ml Worcester sauce

30ml apple cider vinegar

Salt and pepper to taste

Blend all of the ingredients in a food mixer (adding
the liquid ingredients last) until smooth. Marinade your
meat or veggies in the sauce for 4 hours, or overnight
if possible, before cooking on the barbecue.

THE PERFECT VEGGIE BURGER

It's a bold statement to some, but I actually prefer Portobello mushroom burgers to normal beef hamburgers, and especially to traditional 'veggie' burgers! The first time I tried one I knew it was going to make a change to my barbecues at home forever. You can pack a serious amount of veggies into one simple burger, and it's so tasty that veggies and meat-eaters alike will love it. Here is my favourite combination.

Per burger:

Ingredients

1 large Portobello mushroom

½ red pepper, seeds removed and halved horizontally

1 slice large red onion

1 slice beef tomato

3 slim slices avocado

1 slice goat's cheese (the wider the better, so it covers the whole mushroom)

1 burger bun

For the marinade

2 tablespoons oil (I like to use avocado oil)

2 tablespoons balsamic vinegar

2 teaspoons dried rosemary

1 teaspoon chilli flakes

1. Mix your marinade ingredients in a bowl and marinade your vegetables for about an hour.

2. Place your mushroom and pepper on the barbecue first (placing the mushroom face down) for about 5 minutes, before turning them both over and putting the other veggies (except the avocado) on to cook. After a further 5 minutes, flip the veggies over again (except the mushroom) and place the goat's cheese on top of the mushroom to melt. Place your bun on the barbecue to toast also. Cook for a further 2–3 minutes before removing everything from the heat, stacking up the veggies in the bun and adding in the avocado on top.

3. This is perfect to serve with some air-fried sweet potato fries for a healthier alternative to your standard burger and chips!

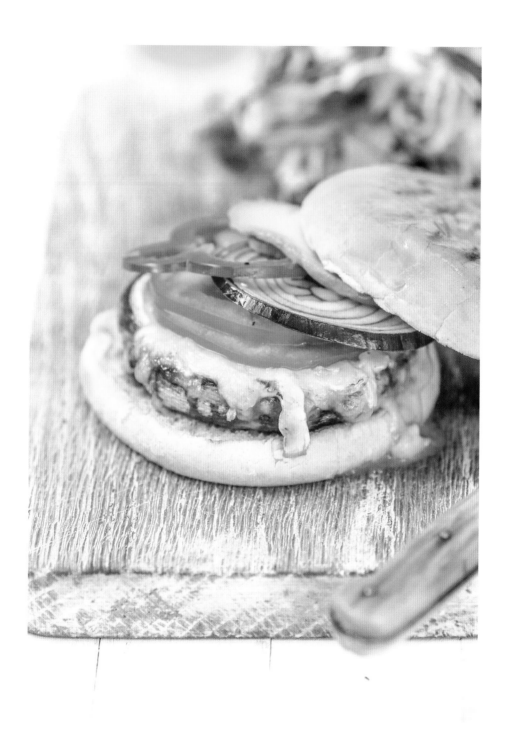

WATERMELON SIDE SALAD

An extension of my favourite watermelon and feta skewers from my quick canapé section (if you liked those, you'll love this!). It's a light, refreshing salad that has a mixture of savoury and sweet flavours that is totally addictive. (Serves 6)

Ingredients
4 mid-sized tomatoes
500g watermelon
200g Feta cheese

For the dressing
10 mint leaves, plus
    extra for garnishing
2 tablespoons olive oil
2 tablespoons red
    wine vinegar
Pinch of chilli flakes

1. Chop the mint leaves very finely, then put all of the dressing ingredients into a bowl and mix well using a fork.
2. Chop the tomatoes into small pieces and the watermelon into bite-sized chunks. Pour over the dressing and crumble the Feta cheese over the top, before tossing gently to combine.
3. Season with salt and pepper and top with a couple of mint leaves for decoration before serving.

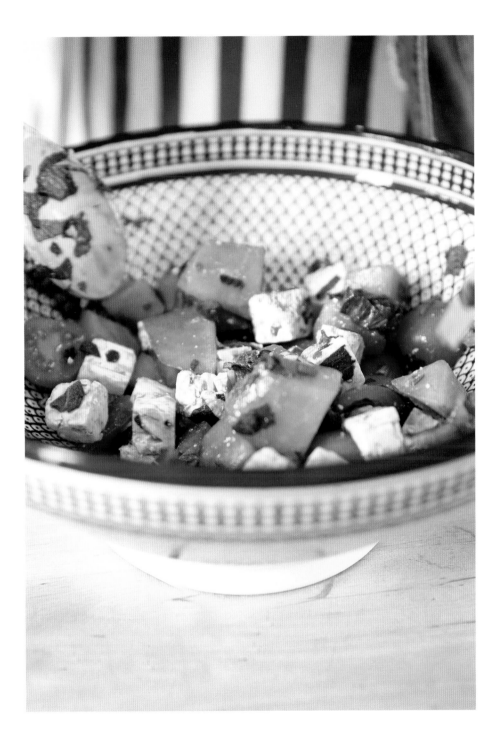

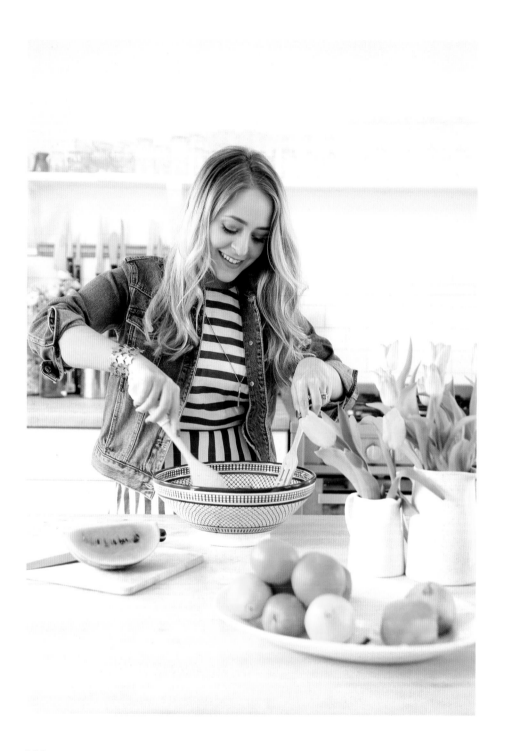

DIY PERI PERI CHICKEN

Peri peri chicken has been one of my favourite barbecue staples for as long as I can remember. It's easy to buy pre-made peri peri marinades and sauces but it's so much tastier to make your own at home, and it only takes a few seconds if you have a food processor or blender (a Nutribullet is perfect for making your own marinades and sauces too!).

(Marinades 6–8 portions of chicken)

Ingredients
4 red chillies
4 cloves garlic
4 sprigs oregano
30g flat-leaf parsley
4 tablespoons olive oil
1 tablespoon smoked paprika
The juice of 1 lemon

1. Top, tail and deseed the chillies, peel the cloves of garlic, remove the leaves of your oregano and discard the stalks and roughly chop the parsley before putting all of the ingredients into a blender to combine.

2. Marinade your chicken in the sauce for 4 hours, or overnight in the fridge, before cooking as normal on the barbecue.

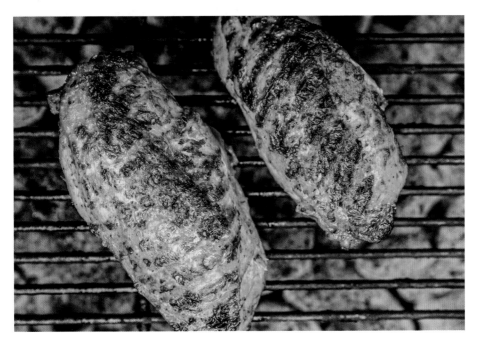

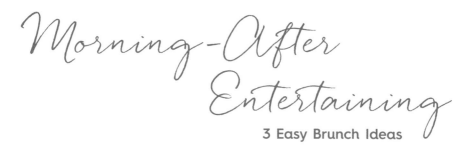

Morning-After Entertaining

3 Easy Brunch Ideas

DEVILLED AVOCADO WITH POACHED EGGS AND CRISPY POLENTA

This recipe is a mismash of some of my favourite breakfasts around London. Polenta (or cornmeal) isn't the most common ingredient these days but it makes for a seriously delicious treat when fried and it's a tasty alternative to ordinary toast. You can buy it dried and ground from supermarkets. This is also a great alternative to a traditional fry up, and it's vegetarian too. It's best to make the polenta a day in advance.

(Per portion, multiply for however many guests you're feeding)

Ingredients

1 ripe avocado

Squeeze of lemon juice

Olive oil

½ fresh red chilli, finely chopped

2 eggs

For the polenta (serves 4–6 when set and baked):

120g ground polenta/ cornmeal

750ml water

1. Boil the water in the kettle and pour into a pan. Add the polenta with some salt and stir in.

2. Continue to stir the polenta as it cooks until it solidifies enough for the edges to pull away from the sides of the pan.

3. Pour the polenta out onto a lined baking tray and allow to cool before refrigerating overnight.

4. When you're ready to cook your breakfast, cut the polenta into squares the size of sliced bread and then cut them from corner to corner into triangles. Place the pieces in a shallow pan with a tiny bit of oil and fry for 7-8 minutes until golden brown on one side, then flip and cook for a further 5 minutes on the other side before removing from the heat.

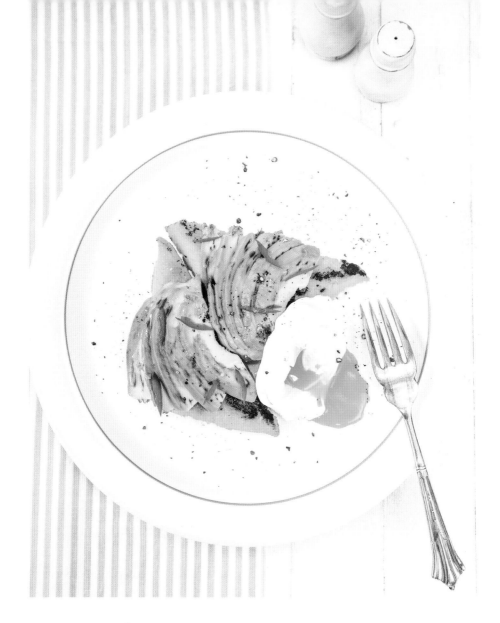

5. In the meantime, peel and mash or fan your avocado(s), adding in a squeeze of lemon, salt and pepper, a drizzle of olive oil and some of that chopped chilli.

6. Soft-poach the eggs in a pan of boiling water. When they are ready, place 2 pieces of crispy polenta on a plate and layer on a generous helping of avocado on top. Finish with the poached eggs and season before serving.

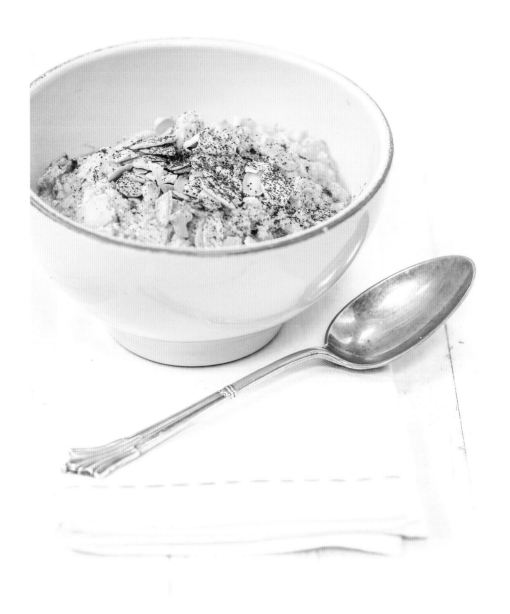

PROPER PORRIDGE

I grew up eating porridge, as it's one of my mum's favourite breakfasts and to me it's one of the ultimate comfort foods. I love making it with coconut milk because it's extra creamy and gives it a really subtle coconut flavour. You can add whatever jams or fruit you like as a topping, but the recipes below are my favourites!

(All porridge recipes serve 4)

Ingredients for basic porridge

200g jumbo porridge oats
1l coconut milk (KoKo is my favourite brand: you want the milk alternative, not traditional 'coconut milk' in a can)

1. Place the oats and milk in a large pan over a medium heat and bring to a gentle simmer.
2. Simmer the porridge for 5–7 minutes, stirring regularly, until the porridge is your favourite consistency. If you need to water it down a little, simply add a splash of cold water.

☆ SPICED ALMOND AND BANANA PORRIDGE

Additional ingredients

2 bananas
30g flaked almonds
½ teaspoon cinnamon, plus extra to serve
½ teaspoon nutmeg
1 teaspoon vanilla extract
Sprinkle of brown sugar (to serve)

1. Peel both of the bananas, mash one and slice the other. When the porridge comes to a simmer, add the mashed banana, along with the almonds, cinnamon, nutmeg and vanilla, and cook with the oats.
2. To serve, add some slices of banana with a sprinkle of ground cinnamon and brown sugar.

✭ MACADAMIA AND MAPLE PORRIDGE

Additional ingredients

4 tablespoons maple syrup, plus extra to serve

2 large handfuls of macadamia nuts

1. Add the maple syrup in to your porridge as you're cooking it.
2. While it is simmering, prepare the macadamia nuts. You can either chop them roughly with a knife, pulse them in a blender or put them in a clean tea towel and break them up with a rolling pin. When the porridge is cooked, stir the nuts in before serving.
3. Top with a drizzle of maple syrup.

✭ ROASTED FIG AND HONEY PORRIDGE

Additional ingredients

4 ripe figs

4 teaspoons pistachio nuts (optional)

4 teaspoons chia seeds

4 tablespoons runny honey

1. Cut the figs into quarters, place them on a baking tray and bake for 15 minutes.
2. Meanwhile, make the porridge and roughly chop the pistachio nuts.
3. Once your porridge is cooked, divide it up between four bowls, pop four pieces of fig on top of each one, sprinkle over the pistachios and chia seeds, and finally drizzle over the honey before serving.

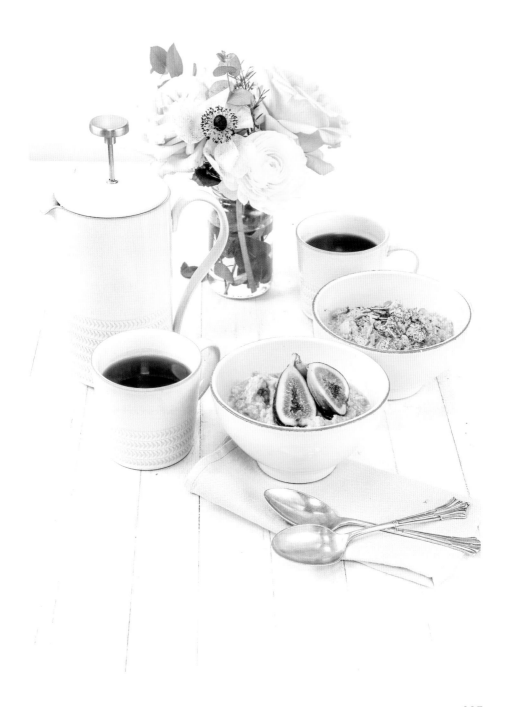

JACK'S BEST BANANA BREAD

My friend Jack is a great cook, but his banana bread is my ultimate favourite thing he's ever made me. It's moist and sticky, with just the right density to make it feel like a treat, yet not overly filling or sickly. It's even better served warm, with a scoop of ice cream!

(Serves 6)

Ingredients

250g plain flour
2 teaspoons baking
   powder
125g butter, softened
235g muscovado
   sugar
400g ripe bananas
100g dark chocolate
1 teaspoon vanilla
   extract
2 tablespoons dark
   rum (optional)
2 eggs

1. Preheat the oven to 180°C/gas mark 4. Line the bottom of a medium loaf tin with greaseproof paper and grease the sides of the tin using the wrapper from your butter.

2. Sift the flour into a bowl and add the baking powder.

3. In another bowl, use an electric whisk to blend together the butter and muscovado sugar.

4. Mash the bananas (the riper the better) in another bowl – you can use a fork or potato masher. Put the dark chocolate into a (clean) tea towel or plastic bag and bash it with a rolling pin to break it up into very small pieces (alternatively you can use dark chocolate chips). Stir it in to the mashed banana, along with the vanilla extract and rum, if using.

5. Beat the eggs into the butter and sugar mixture, introducing a dusting of flour to prevent curdling.

6. Next, fold the chocolate and banana mixture into the sugar mixture and finally fold in the flour. Once fully combined, pour into the loaf tin and bake for 45–50 minutes.

7. Remove the cake from the oven and leave to cool in the tin for 10–15 minutes before using a knife to loosen the sides. You can wait for it to cool, or serve immediately!

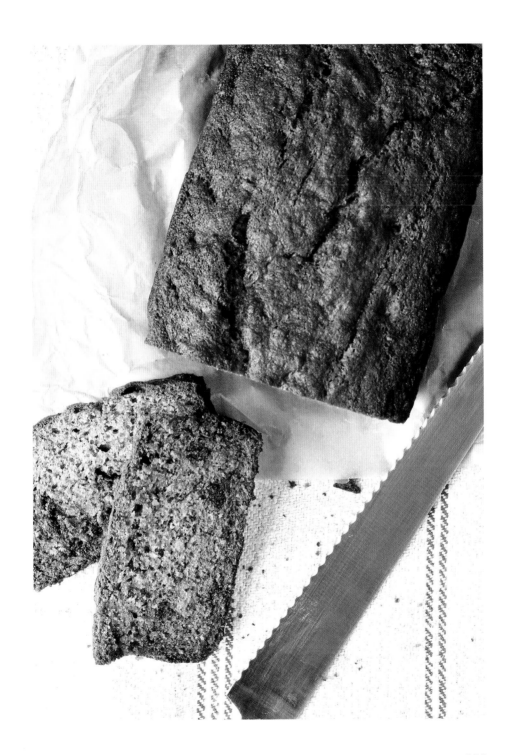

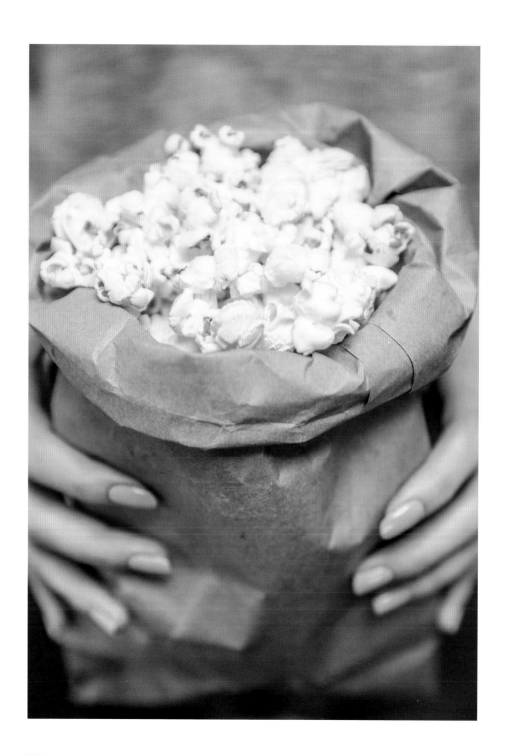

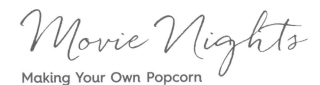

Movie Nights

Making Your Own Popcorn

Popcorn is one of my all-time favourite treats when I go to the cinema, but it's even more delicious made at home and you can get creative with your toppings too. If you've never popped your own corn at home, here's how, and if you want some ideas for tasty flavours and toppings, I've given you my top three!

(All popcorn recipes serve 4)

Ingredients for basic popcorn

6 tablespoons coconut oil (or any other oil that has a high smoke point)

1 cup of popcorn kernels

1. Put the coconut oil into a large pan with a lid, place onto a medium heat and wait for it to melt entirely.
2. Throw in a few popcorn kernels, cover the pan and wait for them to pop.
3. As soon as the kernels pop, add the rest of your corn and shake so they form an even layer over the bottom of the pan. Replace the lid and remove from the heat for 30 seconds.
4. Replace the pan back on the heat. The kernels should start to pop very quickly. As they do, shake the pan gently back and forth to keep the un-popped kernels at the bottom directly on the heat.
5. Keep the lid slightly ajar to let any steam out during the whole process.
6. When the pops start to slow to one every three seconds or so, remove from the pan and pour the popcorn into a large bowl before adding your flavouring of choice!

★ COCONUT MACARON POPCORN

Additional ingredients

3 tablespoons melted
   coconut oil
50g ground almonds
2 teaspoons stevia
1 teaspoon vanilla extract

Combine all the ingredients well in a small bowl then pour over your popcorn, mixing it as you go to ensure it's evenly distributed. As an added extra you can also drizzle over a little melted chocolate!

★ LIME AND CORIANDER POPCORN

Additional ingredients

2 large handfuls coriander
3 tablespoons olive oil
1 fresh lime
1 teaspoon salt

1. Very finely chop the coriander and mix it together in a bowl with the olive oil and juice from the lime.
2. Pour it over your popcorn, mixing or shaking as you go to make sure it's evenly distributed.
3. Finally, add the salt little by little, mixing well.

★ ROSEMARY AND PARMESAN POPCORN

Additional ingredients

2 cloves garlic
2 sprigs fresh rosemary
2 teaspoons sea salt
3 tablespoons olive oil
100g Parmesan cheese

1. Using a pestle and mortar, crush the garlic cloves, rosemary leaves (discard the stalks) and sea salt together. Add the olive oil and continue to grind everything together for a couple of minutes.
2. Pour the oil mixture over the popcorn, mixing it in as you go to get a more even distribution.
3. Grate the Parmesan over the popcorn, again mixing as you go.

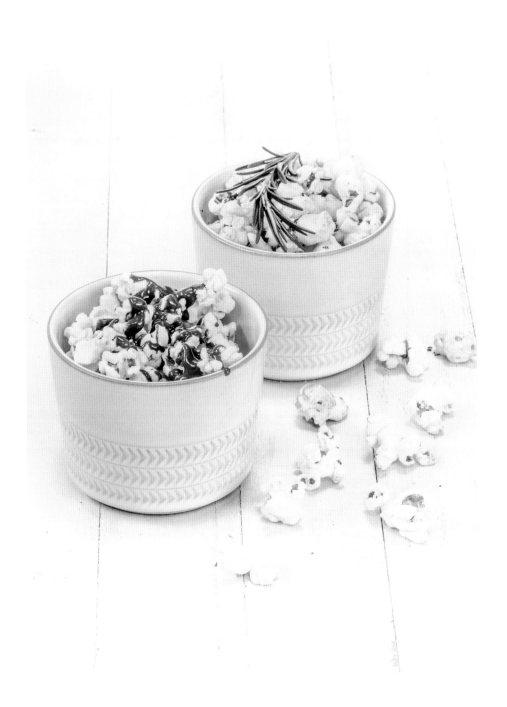

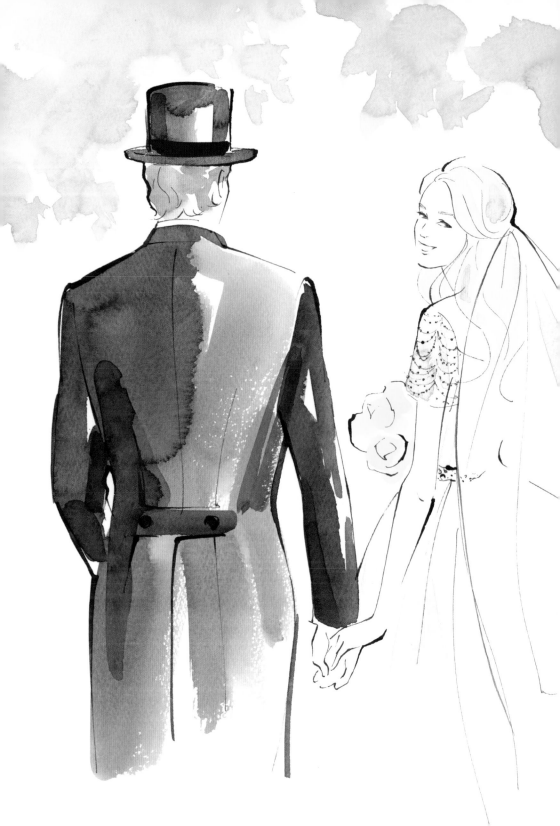

Wedding Belles

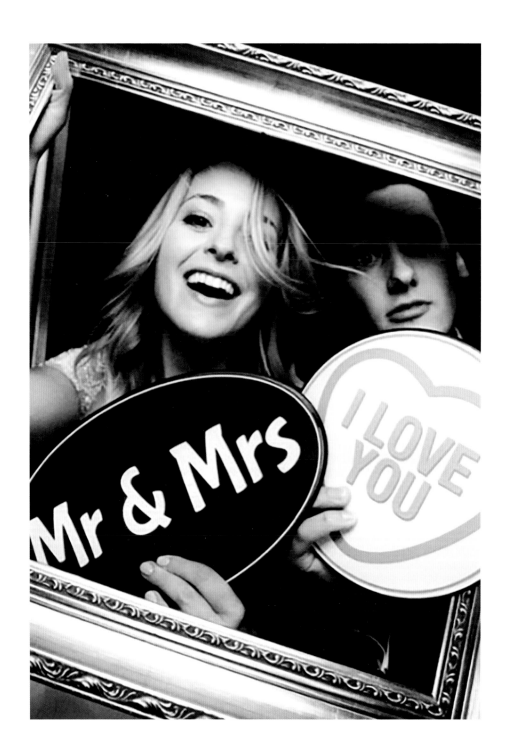

Introduction

Weddings are one of my favourite occasions to dress up for. There's something very special about celebrating a wedding. It's the most romantic of events and I am always really excited not just to see what the bride's wearing, but what everyone else is wearing too. This chapter is all about weddings, from what to wear yourself to modern-day wedding etiquette and some imaginative wedding gift ideas if you want to go off the wedding list.

What to Wear

Beach wedding

Beach weddings tend to have a bit more of a casual, boho vibe than traditional weddings, so you can get away with more casual styles, and relaxed maxi dresses work really well. If any part of the day is actually on the beach itself, think carefully about your footwear. If you really want to wear heels, go for wedges to make it easier for yourself, but if you go for a flowing maxi dress, you can get away with flat sandals that will be easier to walk in and more comfortable too. A large, floppy hat also makes a practical and stylish addition to shade your face from the sun.

Country wedding

For country weddings, it's best to go for something that isn't floor-length to avoid grass stains on the hem of your dress. Try to opt for wedges or sturdy heels to avoid sinking into the soft grass or falling on uneven ground. It's worth taking a stole, jacket or cover-up for the evening, as marquees tend to get cold.

City wedding

City weddings generally have a more modern vibe, so more fashion-forward designs look great. Go for a playsuit or a bright-coloured dress with killer heels. You won't have to negotiate your way over grass, sand or pebbles and there's unlikely to be much walking.

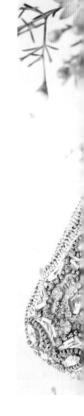

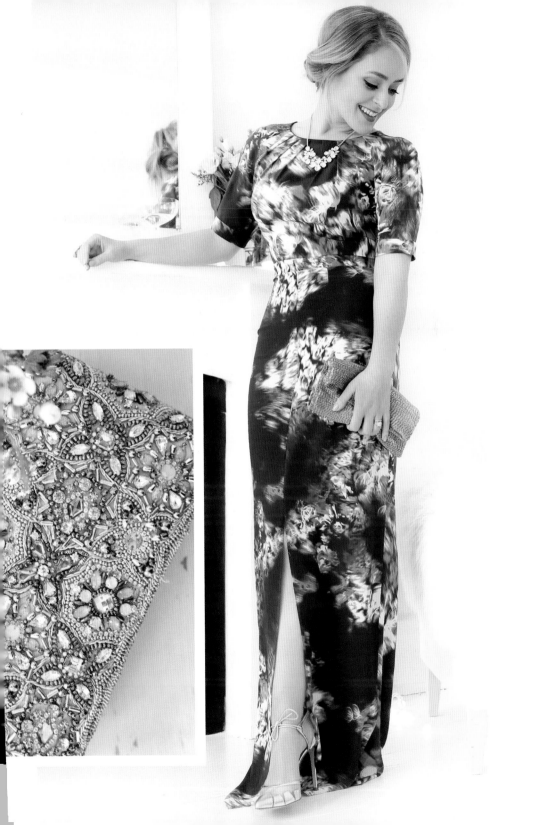

Church/traditional wedding

For more traditional church weddings you might want to think about covering up a little more than you otherwise would. It's traditional and respectful to cover your shoulders in church, but not totally essential. For the most traditional weddings (especially in the UK), one of the best things is getting the opportunity to wear a hat. Just remember, you're not supposed to remove your hat at the reception until the mother of the bride has and gentlemen traditionally keep their jackets on until the groom has removed his.

Winter wedding

It can be tricky to find the right balance between warmth and style at winter weddings, as it's hard to make thick winter coats look formal and feminine. Faux-fur stoles make a nice addition to winter wedding attire and classic black leather gloves also help to keep the look more formal even when you're bundled up. If you want to go for opaque black tights, make sure you pair them with closed-toe shoes.

Casual wedding

For more casual weddings, you don't want to be overdressed, especially if the bride herself isn't wearing a traditional gown – there's nothing worse than upstaging the bride at her own wedding!

Dos and don'ts when dressing for weddings

DON'T wear white or cream unless you're part of the bridal party and the bride wants you to!

DON'T wear a very long, formal dress if you know the wedding has a casual setting (it might end up being almost as formal as the bride's!).

DO bring a change of shoes if you can, especially for all-day weddings if you're wearing high heels.

DO pack a compact umbrella in your bag if you know the wedding's going to be outside.

Wedding Etiquette

It can sound old-fashioned talking about 'etiquette', but weddings are one of the most important days in many people's lives and with social-media culture changing the way we share our lives, it's important to be aware of what's acceptable in modern wedding etiquette.

When to arrive

Being 'fashionably late' doesn't really apply to weddings unless you're the bride. The bride usually arrives around fifteen minutes late for the ceremony. It's the ultimate wedding faux-pas to arrive after the bride, so play it safe and aim to arrive fifteen minutes before the ceremony is due to start.

When and what to share

In the culture of social media, it comes as second nature to share everything instantly online, but when it comes to weddings, take it as a general rule not to share any images of the couple, the dress or any 'spoilers' from the wedding before the couple have shared it themselves, unless they have specifically asked you to share your images using a hashtag or shared album. That way you're not risking offending anyone, and are probably enjoying the day and 'living in the moment' a little more!

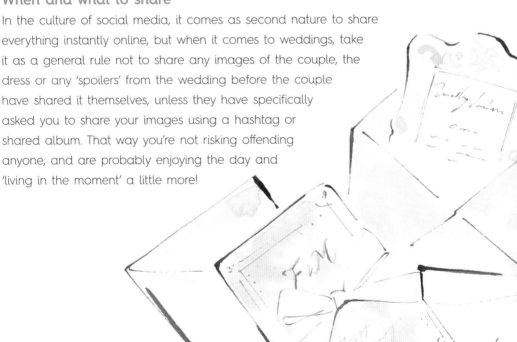

What to spend

When it comes to gifts, there isn't really a set amount to spend per person. Gifting is usually all about the 'thought' but when it comes to weddings, there's often a gift list so it can take that element of thought away. I personally think off-the-list gifts are much more special, so if you don't have a huge amount to spend, consider going off-list and take inspiration from some of my ideas below.

Who to thank

Writing thank-you letters is the done thing when it comes to weddings, but sometimes it's tricky to know who to thank. In the old days, the bride's parents used to pay for the wedding, so they were the main people to thank, but nowadays most couples foot the bill themselves, or have some financial help from both sets of parents. The best way to know who to thank is to look at the invitation to see who has formally invited you to the wedding. Also take note of the location of the reception. If it's hosted at someone's house, you should thank them, too. As a general rule, I write thank-you notes to the couple and both sets of parents the week after the wedding.

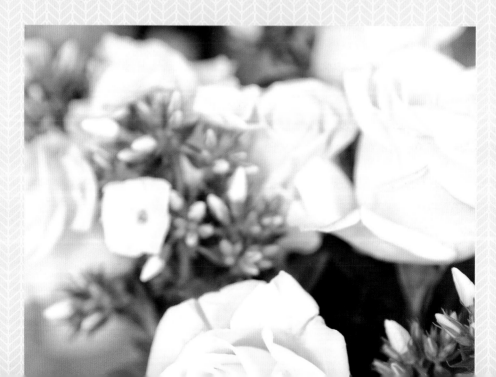

DIY Wedding Gifts

You don't have to spend a fortune to give the couple in question a really personal, special, one-off wedding present. The following are my favourite personalised DIY gifts for newlyweds if you want to give them something extra special that they'll be able to treasure for years to come, without breaking the bank!

PERSONALISED PICNIC BASKET

This idea is perfect for foodie couples as you're not only giving them a lovely personalised picnic basket, but you can fill it with all of their favourite treats! All you need to do is buy a plain picnic basket from a craft or hardware store, cut out some initial stencils and spray-paint the couple's initials on the front. I like to decorate the rest of the basket with ribbons and/or embellishments (depends on the couple), and you can then use ribbons to tie in the cutlery and a few plates. I like to use mismatching vintage cake plates for this, which you can pick up in antique shops and flea markets very cheaply. Then you can fill it with whatever you think the couple might like. Champagne and chocolates make a good start but just remember not to put anything perishable in there as a lot of couples don't open all their gifts until they return from their honeymoon.

You will need
* A picnic basket
* Initial stencils (can easily be made from A4 paper)
* Spray paint in colour of your choice
* Ribbons to decorate and secure cutlery
* Tissue paper
* Treats to put inside!

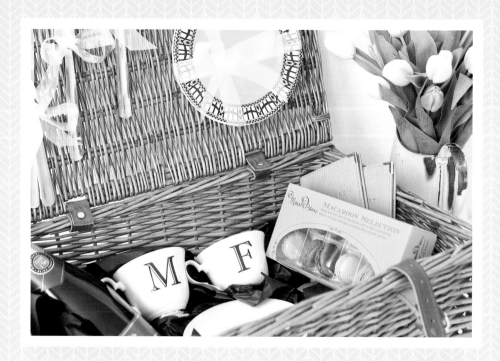

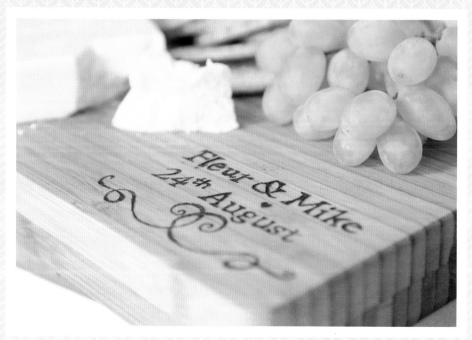

PERSONALISED CHOPPING BOARD

This DIY project is perfect for foodie couples or homebodies. It's something they'll probably end up using every day because it's really practical, but being personalised, it's special at the same time. You can get creative and freehand draw your design, or if you want a more uniform design or you're not the best artist, you can print off your design and trace it on!

You will need
* A wooden chopping board
* A wood-burning set (available online or from craft shops)
* A pencil

Optional
* A printout of what you want to engrave (you can use an image, pattern, text etc)
* Graphite paper (again, available online or from craft shops)
* Sellotape

Start by drawing your design onto the board in pencil. If you want to trace the design, print it off first and use your graphite paper to transfer the design onto the wood (tape it all in place first to avoid it shifting around whilst you're working).

Next, heat up your wood-burning tool and draw over your design with it, burning it into the wood. This will turn the wood black wherever you touch so be careful to do this neatly (and also be careful not to burn yourself!).

HIS 'N' HERS SHARPIE MUGS

This cute DIY gift idea is one of the most affordable options, but still a thoughtful personalised gift. You can do a set of two mugs, or more depending on what kind of message you want to personalise it with!

You will need
* Plain white mugs
* A Sharpie in a colour of your choice
* An A4 sheet of large white sticky labels to make stencils

Start by printing off the initials of your couple onto your white sticky labels. Cut around the letters carefully to create stencils, then stick them onto your mugs. Then take your Sharpie and start drawing different-sized dots on the mug, focusing on the area immediately around the stencils, and diffusing outwards. Leave the ink to dry for half an hour, then draw over the dots again to intensify the colour. At this point you can also add a message on the bottom of the mug (the wedding date, your name, an in-joke etc!). Once the second coat of ink is dry, remove the sticky stencils and place your mug into the oven. Turn the oven on to 150°C for thirty minutes, then turn it off and wait for the oven to completely cool before removing your mug. This helps to 'bake' the colour on and makes sure it stays for longer!

Tip Don't forget to include a note letting the couple know to hand-wash the mugs! Putting them in the dishwasher will cause the ink to fade more quickly.

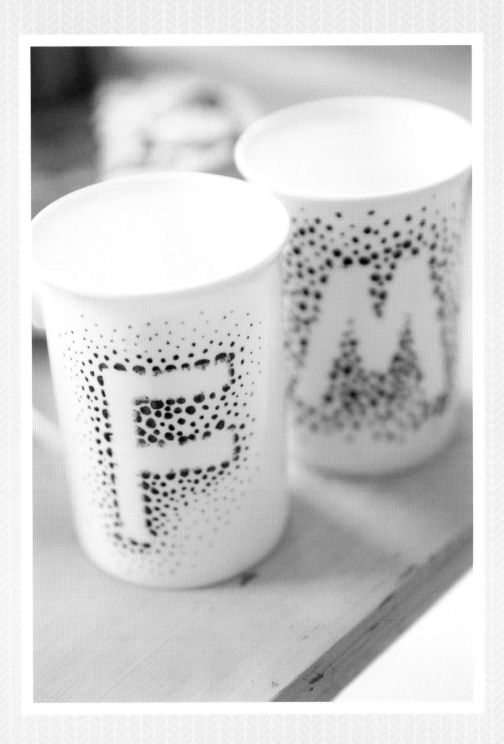

POLAROID PEG & STRING FRAME

One of the nicest personalised gift ideas is to use images from the couple's wedding. Professional photographs usually take at least a week or two to come through, so if you make a DIY gift using Polaroid photos from the day, it's extra special for the couple as it will probably be their first hard-copy images of the occasion.

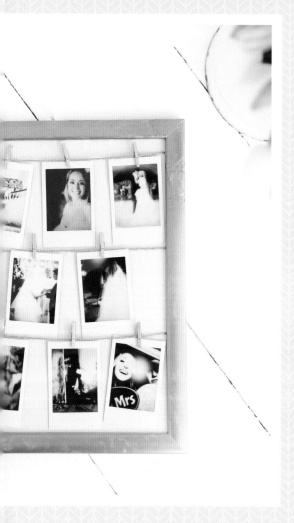

You will need
* A4 picture frame
* A4 pearlised paper
* Sellotape
* Brown string
* 6 miniature pegs
* Polaroids from the wedding day
* A Sharpie (this is optional if you want to write captions on the pictures!)

Start by pre-making the frame. You can get creative with this part, but one of my favourite things to do is use an A4 frame, remove the glass and mount some brown string running in three lines horizontally over pearlised paper. I then place two mini pegs on each line of string and hang a miniature Polaroid from each. It's so simple, really affordable and is guaranteed to be a hit with the newlyweds.

5 of the Best
Wedding Gift Ideas

If you don't want to get crafty, but you still want to buy something for the couple off the list so it's a surprise, here are my top five wedding gift ideas. A few of these are things my husband and I were bought by thoughtful guests at our wedding and others are gifts I've bought for others that have gone down really well in the past.

A honeymoon experience

The perfect present for a couple you know very well, or for a newlywed family member, organising a surprise experience for the couple while they are on their honeymoon is an opportunity to make their trip even more memorable. A lot of honeymoon companies now offer the chance to gift money towards a honeymoon, or book excursions of the couple's choice while they're away, but essentially that's the same thing as giving money. I personally like to ring ahead to their destination hotel and speak to the concierge about activities in the area. If it's a couple I know well, it's easy to gauge what activities or extras will interest them, so I go ahead and organise it as a surprise for when they arrive. Whether it's an excursion, a special meal during their stay or even champagne and chocolates upon arrival, it makes for a more memorable gift than one bought from a gift list.

A post-wedding treat

Getting home from your honeymoon can often be a huge downer. After all the excitement of the wedding and the honeymoon, most couples arrive home to a huge workload waiting for them after having time off, and a depleted bank balance. I love the idea of getting a couple a lovely experience for them to enjoy once all the fanfare wears off. Whether it's a voucher to a fancy restaurant, a night's stay in a smart hotel for a weekend away or tickets to the theatre, it's so nice to have a treat like that waiting for you when you come home.

History of love mugs

This was my personal favourite gift that my husband and I received from a friend when we got married and it's become something of a go-to wedding gift for me to buy for couples ever since, as we use them every single day! My favourites from Susan Rose China have hand-drawn personalised lettering and are made from beautiful fine bone china.

His 'n' hers dressing gowns

It might sound a little cheesy, but another great wedding gift that is guaranteed to get used on a daily basis is a set of his 'n' hers dressing gowns. There are loads of different websites that offer embroidery services on towelling goods. You can go for a simple 'Mr' and 'Mrs' or get more personal with their names or nicknames.

Personalised passport covers

Gifts that you can take with you and use on your honeymoon are a lovely treat for a wedding present and even more so if they are personalised. Matching passport covers are a lovely idea for a honeymoon-appropriate wedding gift, made even better if you can get them personalised. My favourite place for small leather

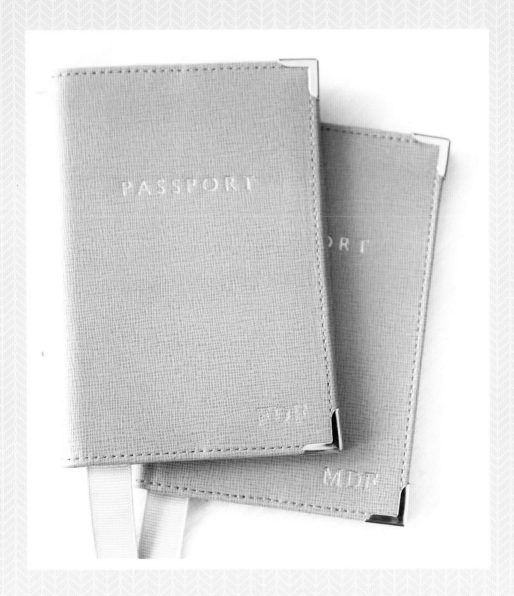

goods like this is Aspinal of London as they aren't overpriced and they offer in-house personalisation that they can usually do while you wait. If you don't think passport covers are up their street, they also do lovely luggage tags too. If either party is changing their name, it also makes a lovely gift as it will probably be their first time using their new initials!

the Art of Giving

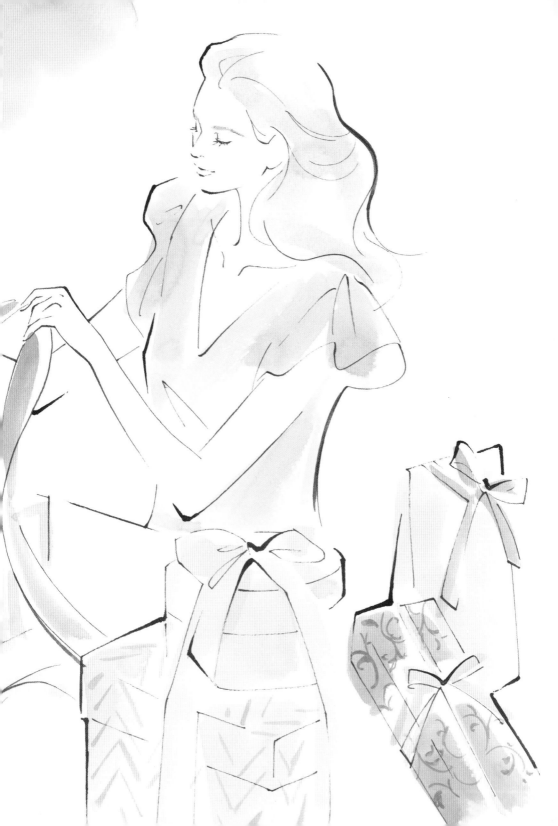

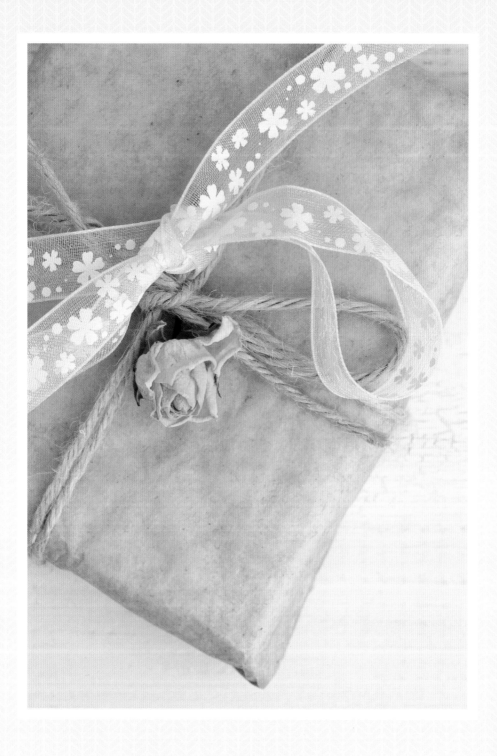

DIY Gifts: Luxe on a Budget

Some DIY gifts are pretty cringeworthy, I have to admit – I'm pretty sure we've all been there when it comes to receiving awful home-made presents and having to try really hard to pretend we love them, but good DIY gifts show that luxe does not have to mean expensive. When you get it right with DIY gifts they can be one of the most thoughtful and well-received options, as it shows you've put a lot of time, effort and thought into it. I also love making DIY gifts as you can make them in big batches and customise each for whoever you're giving it to! These are four of my favourite DIY presents that won't cost you an arm and a leg, and are well worth putting the time in to make them.

RHUBARB GIN IN WASHI-TAPE BOTTLES

Infusing your own gin is a great idea for friends and family alike. Sloe gin works really well for Christmas, but my personal favourite is rhubarb-infused gin, which is great for summer birthdays or bringing to summer barbecues or dinner parties. As an added touch I like to decorate the bottles with washi tape. If you've never used washi tape before, it's a multi-use decorative tape that can be used to customise or decorate pretty much anything! You can pick it up really easily online or in some stationery and craft stores.

You will need

* 1 large jar with a tight-fitting lid. If you're making a bigger batch of gin it's a good idea to purchase a large Kilner jar to store the gin in while it infuses, then divide it between smaller bottles to give away
* 1 empty, clean bottle – you can reuse one or buy one
* 400g fresh rhubarb – as ripe as you can find, the pinker the better!
* 120g sugar
* 1 fresh lemon
* 700ml gin
* Some washi tape in your chosen design – you might want a few different styles to get creative with your bottle!
* A permanent marker pen
* A selection of ribbon

Step 1 Top and tail the rhubarb before chopping it into small chunks and placing it at the bottom of your jar.

Step 2 Add the sugar and the juice of your lemon (squeeze it through your fingers to catch any pips!).

Step 3 Add the gin, close the lid and shake well.

Step 4 Leave the gin for at least two weeks (longer if possible), shaking it every now and again to encourage the sugar to fully dissolve.

Step 5 Decorate the bottle using washi tape and personalise it with your marker pen.

Step 6 Next, use a funnel and a sieve to carefully pour the gin into your bottle, removing the rhubarb. Replace the lid tightly and tie a ribbon of your choice around the neck of the bottle.

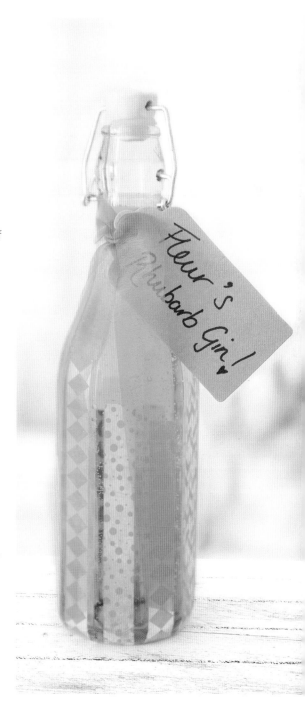

DIY CAMERA STRAP

This gift is perfect for budding photographers and bloggers, as it's a nice way to customise your camera. If you've always got the strap around your neck or shoulder, it looks a bit smarter and makes the camera more comfortable to carry too. It is really simple and easy to make.

You will need

* 1 scarf – you can use an old one or buy one especially for this if there's a certain style you have in mind. Smaller, rectangular scarves (rather than square) work the best and silk scarves also look really nice
* 2 slim keyring clips, or split-rings (available from craft shops)
* A stapler

Step 1 Loop the end of your scarf through the ring of your clip or split-ring and fold it back on itself.

Step 2 Staple the point where you want your knot to be a few times (crossing over your staples is a good idea for extra security) You also want to leave a little extra bit of the tail of the scarf above your staples, then knot the scarf to cover up your staples and further secure the strap. Repeat on the other end of the scarf.

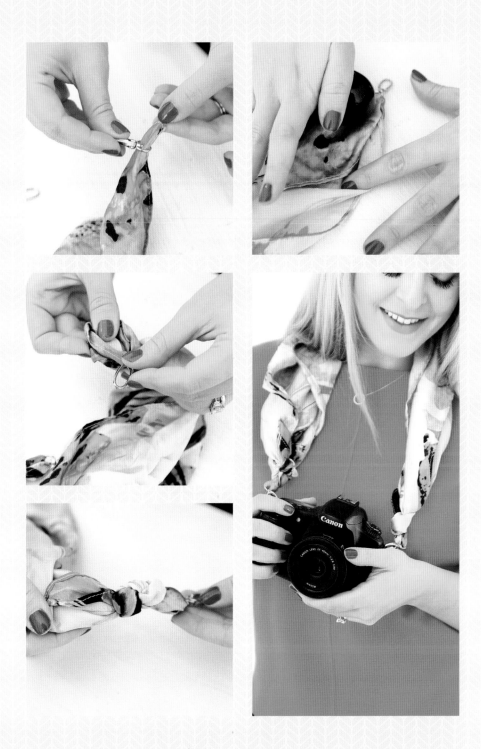

MARBLED ESPRESSO MUGS

You can choose the colours to personalise these pretty marbled mugs with. My personal favourite is a rainbow of pastel colours, but black works really well for a simple, chic look or a more masculine feel. The technique for creating these uses nail polish and is the same as marble nail art!

You will need
* Simple white espresso mugs (with saucers if possible – they look cute in matching pairs)
* Nail polish in colours of your choice (preferably not quick-drying formulas)
* A few cocktail sticks
* A medium-sized plastic Tupperware container

Step 1 Fill your Tupperware container ¾ full with very hot water.

Step 2 Add a few drops of your chosen nail polish colour onto the surface of the water (drop it onto the water from as close to the surface as you can, otherwise the polish will sink to the bottom).

Step 3 Moving as quickly as possible so the polish doesn't dry, swirl the polish around on the surface of the water, then dip your mug into the water.

Step 4 Place your mug on a paper towel to dry and it's done!

Step 5 If you want to change colours, change your water up between each one.

Step 6 Make sure you let the recipient know that the mugs aren't dishwasher safe, in order to preserve the design.

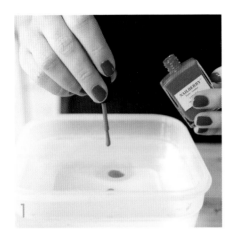

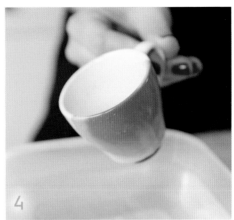

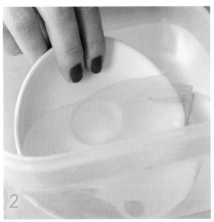

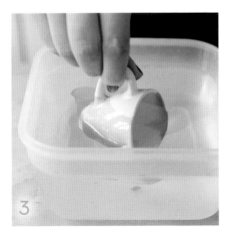

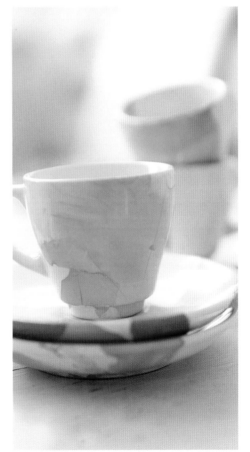

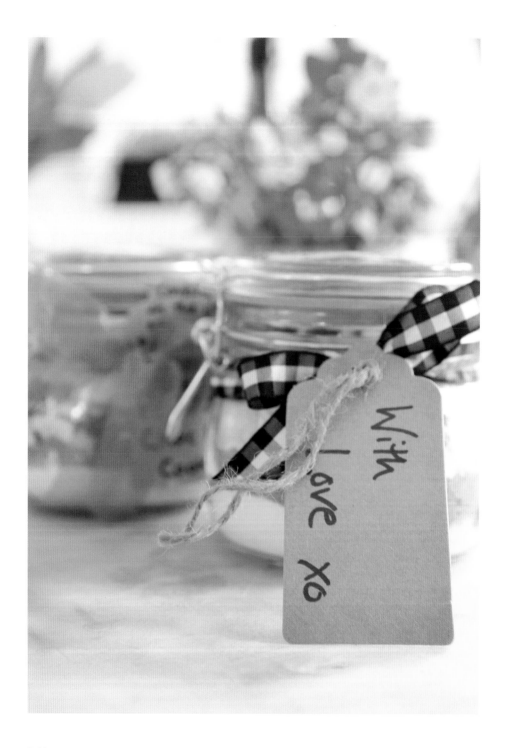

PEANUT AND CHOC-CHIP COOKIE JAR

Bake-it-yourself jars have become really popular over the past few years, but there's no point in buying them from a shop when you can so easily make a DIY version and personalise both the packaging and the recipe. You can adapt this idea for any of your favourite recipes but this peanut and choc-chip cookie recipe is my personal favourite.

Allergy Advice: For allergens, (including cereals containing gluten,) see asterisked ingredients

You will need

- ✷ A medium-sized Kilner jar
- ✷ Ribbon to decorate
- ✷ A large brown gift tag
- ✷ A large brown label
- ✷ 160g plain flour
- ✷ 110g brown sugar
- ✷ 50g granulated sugar
- ✷ 1 teaspoon ground cinnamon
- ✷ ½ teaspoon baking soda
- ✷ Pinch of salt
- ✷ 75g roughly chopped peanuts*
- ✷ 150g milk chocolate chips

Step 1 Layer up the ingredients into the jar, as they are listed to the left. You want to do this gently, evening out each ingredient as you go to create distinct layers that you can see through the sides of the jar.

Step 2 Seal the jar carefully and tie a ribbon around the neck.

Step 3 Write on your label the name of the recipe, the name of the person you're giving it too, or even your own name if you want (e.g. 'Fleur's Yummy Peanut Cookies').

Step 4 On the brown tag, write the cooking instructions and additional ingredients needed, as follows:

'Combine all of the ingredients in the jar with 110g butter and 1 egg. Roll into small balls and place on a baking sheet before baking at 180°C/gas mark 4 for 10 minutes. Remove and place on a wire rack for 5 minutes before serving warm.'

DIY Wrapping Paper

Beautiful wrapping paper makes a gift extra special, regardless of what's inside, and if you've hand-made that wrapping paper it's even more special. I personally love getting creative with my wrapping, whether it's making my own designs or trying out different ideas for unusual packaging. These are my top five favourite ways to personalise my wrapping paper and add a little extra touch to any present I'm giving.

Editorial wrap

Make use of your favourite magazine editorial after you've read it by using the pages to wrap a present. This makes it really easy to customise your wrapping for each person, and newspapers work equally as well. Use the travel section for those with itchy feet, the beauty section for makeup addicts and glossy fashion editorials for fashionistas. You can then decorate with eclectic mismatched ribbon or make a decorative multi-strand bow using other pages from the same publication.

Tape it up

Use Japanese washi tape to decorate plain brown paper in a pattern of your choice. You can also use it to keep the paper together like normal tape, but conceal it with the rest of your pattern, or cut out smaller shapes and use them to make a pattern.

Chalk board

Use black paper to wrap your presents, then get a white chalk marker pen to customise the paper. You can either write a message on it once it's already wrapped or draw a pattern onto the paper before you start wrapping. You can also get coloured chalk pens, which make a fun alternative for children's gifts. I love decorating this with brown paper string to continue the more basic theme.

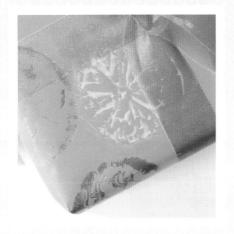

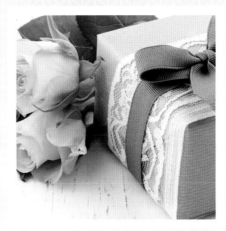

Citrus stamp

A slightly messier alternative to drawing a pattern is to use citrus fruit to make a stamp. I love doing this in the spring or summertime. Take some plain paper (I prefer lime green paper) and cut a lemon in half. Remove the pips and use a sharp knife to cut slightly into each segment to make the lines more pronounced (similar to cutting a grapefruit but not all the way down!) , then dry off the surface of the lemon before dipping it in paint and stamping it all over the green paper. I use one side of the lemon to stamp yellow paint, then the other side to stamp orange paint. Wait for the paper to dry fully before wrapping your present in it and finish it off with a big pink ribbon.

Little brown box

If you're looking for a creative way to wrap jewellery or other small gifts, don't throw away the centre roll of you wrapping paper! Cut it into small 10-cm (4-inch) sections. Flatten each one, then fold in the two sides of each end into a neat curve, closing it up. Wrap your gift in tissue paper, pop it inside, then tape each end and decorate it with ribbon, string, tape or stickers. You can also use the inside of toilet rolls for the same effect!

How to Wrap the Perfect Present

It may sound really basic, but there's actually quite an art to wrapping the perfect present! Follow my steps below for gifts that look like they've been professionally gift-wrapped.

* Cut your paper to the right size. You want the paper to reach all the way around your gift, with an inch to spare. At the ends you need to have just under the full depth of your present on each side. This will make sure you don't have any added bulk at the ends, and can easily fold them neatly.

* Fold the edges. Once you've folded in your edges, make sure you fold over any ends that are showing for the neatest finish.

* Use double-sided tape. It's not just for Blue Peter projects! Using double-sided tape means you don't have to have tape showing on the outside. Place it on the underside of your fold as close as possible to the edge of the paper so you don't have any loose edges, then press down firmly to secure.

* Wrapping soft items: If you're wrapping a soft gift such as a scarf or an item of clothing, put a square of cardboard underneath it, fold it neatly then wrap it around the cardboard. This will ensure your gift is not only much neater looking, but also easier to wrap as well.

* DIY bows: Ribbon can be pricey and the cost can quickly add up if you've got a lot of gifts to wrap. Try making your own ribbons from excess wrapping, folding over the strips of paper and taping them down at the end.

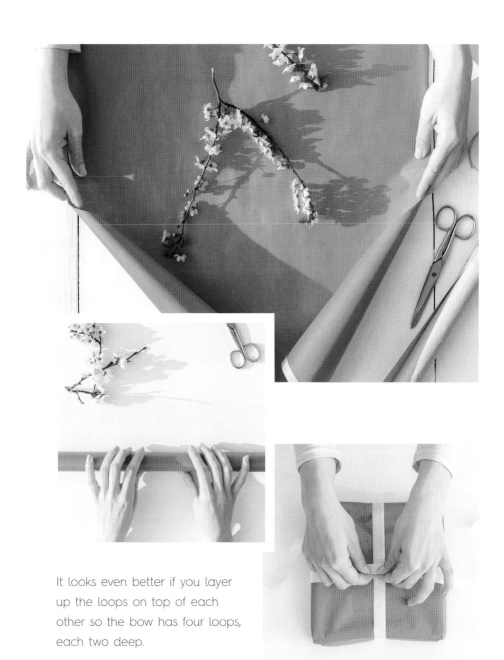

It looks even better if you layer up the loops on top of each other so the bow has four loops, each two deep.

Luxe Gift Ideas
for Everyone

If you're not into making your own presents or don't have the time, the following gifts are my top go-to recommendations year on year. Obviously this list is not exhaustive. If you want more recommendations I make Christmas gift guides every year on my YouTube channel so I would recommend taking a look at those for further inspiration.

FOR HIM

For the man who has everything

My husband is one of those men who buys pretty much anything he has his eyes on within a few weeks, days or hours (!) of deciding he wants it, so I struggle to choose both smaller and more substantial gifts for him. One thing I've found works every time is a cool, token gadget. Obviously these change every year but whatever newly released miniature remote-controlled helicopter, drone, portable speakers or pocket-sized gizmo has just hit the shops is a sure-fire hit for the man who has everything.

For the adventurer

A scratch map makes a great gift for travel-loving guys. It's a large wall-hung map of the world where you scratch off each country you've been to (with the end goal of visiting them all!).

For the gamer

There is a huge variety of gaming gifts depending on which games they are into. A couple of gifts that are bound to be a hit regardless of their choice in games are anti-fatigue glasses (with lenses that block out blue light, glare and UV) and, if you're feeling a bit more flush (and probably if you don't live with the recipient!), a gaming chair is also a great gift. You can get specific ones for different games or more generic ones. They vary in price quite a lot, but are a great choice for true gamers.

For the hipster

A beautifully framed print of their favourite album artwork, a rare vinyl for their collection or (if they have a stereotypical 'hipster beard') a beard-trimming kit all make great gifts.

For the fashion-conscious man

You can't go wrong with a good leather hold-all, especially for a fashionable gent. If you go for real leather, look for a denser textured leather with heavy-duty zips and it's more likely to age well over time.

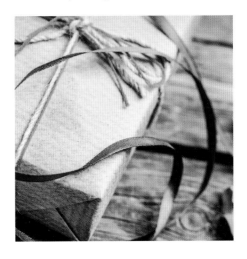

FOR HER

For the beauty addict
A personalised makeup bag makes an amazing gift for
beauty lovers. You can get some cool clear plastic ones
with slots to insert pictures in, or you can get one printed.

For the fashionista
When it comes to fashion lovers, you can't go far wrong
with a voucher for their favourite store, but I personally
hate buying people vouchers or gifting money, so maybe
go for a personal shopping experience instead! I love
doing this in Topshop. It's free to book and you can put
a voucher behind the till for them to contribute towards
their shopping.

For the homebody
Anthropologie is my favourite shop when it comes to
buying gifts for homebodies. They have so many beautiful
home gifts, but my favourites are their Capri Blue candles.
They come in beautiful jars with metal lids that can be
reused for storage when they're finished (see my section
on candles to see how to do this).

For the traveller

A personalised luggage tag makes a great gift for any traveller. Aspinal of London make the best quality ones that are still value for money and they offer an embossing service for a small fee.

For the keen cook

There are many restaurants that offer one-day or half-day cookery courses for not too much money. They're never usually that serious and end up with you getting the chance to eat the fruits of your labour all together over a glass of wine at the end of the course, so it's a fun activity to do with the person you're buying the gift for. I was given a great chocolate-making course at Hotel Chocolat in London's Borough Market.

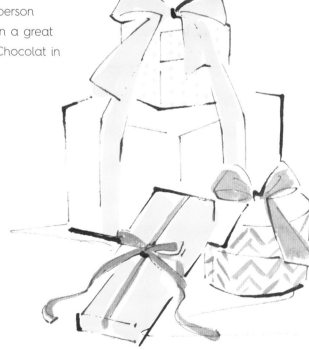

My Guide to Last-Minute Gift Buying

Write a list

It may seem obvious, but write a list of who you need to shop for before you head out on your shopping mission, along with any ideas you may have for what to buy each person and which shops you want to prioritise to get all your shopping done.

Set a budget

After completing your list, set a budget for each person, based on a share of your total budget, and make a note of it next to their name.

Do your research

Before setting a foot out of the door, do your research online for anything you know you might want to get. Not only are items often cheaper on the internet, but it will also save you having to carry any heavier items around with you when shopping. Last-minute shopping before Christmas can also work in your favour as a lot of shops start their sales the week before Christmas now, so you might be able to bag some bargains.

Shop online first

If you see something you want to get in a shop, but it's a little over budget, it's worth checking on your phone if it's available cheaper anywhere else. Always remember to check delivery dates, though! At busy times of year, delivery dates may be delayed and there's nothing worse than receiving a gift in the post the day after you wanted to give it.

Get there early

If you have a full day available for your last-minute shopping, try to get out into the shops as early as possible so that they are as orderly as they are ever going to be that day. It'll be easier to navigate the shelves if they are better organised and also a much nicer shopping experience if there are fewer people in the shops.

Look for last-minute sales

Before you leave the house, it's worth having a look online for any seasonal or last-minute sales that you may need a voucher for. These are rife around Christmas and often associated with magazines so it's worth having a scan of those too. They usually offer 25–30 per cent off your entire purchase, so it's well worth doing if you're trying to stick within a set budget.

Always ask if the shop offers gift-wrapping

If shops offer gift-wrapping, it's often free so well worth doing if you're short on time as you won't have to spend time wrapping it yourself.

Last resorts

There are always those final two or three gifts that you're unable to find and if you're running out of time it can make things really stressful! If in doubt, opt for food gifts (chocolates, cheese or wine) or gift vouchers. It lacks imagination but will always be appreciated if chosen correctly.

Keep comfortable

If you're uncomfortable, hungry or tired, you're going to be less efficient and more likely to give up before finishing your list. Make sure you wear comfortable shoes and stop for a coffee or food break when you need one!

Fashion Directory

H&M, trouser
Topshop, vest
ASOS, Moyna clutch
Valentino, heels

Page 87
Day:
Karen Millen, leather trouser
Urban Outfitters, Light Before
    Dark jacket
H&M, tshirt
Saint Laurent, loafers
Night Additions:
Karen Millen, leather trouser
Reiss, blouse
Zara, heels
Reiss, clutch bag

Page 88
Day:
Topshop, boots
Oasis, jean
The Outnet, Iris & Ink jumper
Orelia, jewellery
Night Additions:
Topshop, boots
Reiss, leather jacket
French Connection, dress
Necklace, stylists own
YSL, bag

Page 89
Net-a-Porter, Alice +
    Olivia jumpsuit
Bionda Castana, mules
Astley Clarke, necklace

Page 90
The Outnet, Iris & Ink
    leather jacket
Zoe Karssen, tee

Page 93
Clockwise from top left
Topshop, jumpsuit
Belt, stylists own

The Outnet, Iris & Ink shirt
French Connection, skirt
YSL, bag
Topshop, shirt
Banana Republic, necklace

Page 95
The Outnet, W118 By
Walter Baker top
Needle & Thread, skirt
Chelsea Paris, heels
Astley Clarke, rings
Carat, X ring

Page 98
Zara, heels

Page 110
Carat, jewellery
Net-a-Porter, Alice +
    Olivia dress

Page 115
Carat, X ring
Astley Clarke, rings
Orelia, O ring
J Crew, star ring
Susan Caplan, pearl
    necklace
Orelia, O necklace
J Crew, bracelet

Page 117
Gianvito Rossi heels,
    Fleur's own
Carat, jewellery

Luxe at Home
Page 120
French Connection, trouser
Urban Outfitters,
    Cooperative polo-neck
Carat London, ring

Page 123
French Connection, trouser
Urban Outfitters,
    Cooperative polo-neck
Carat London, ring
Faux fur stole, stylist's own
Valentino, green bag

Perfect Party Food
Page 176
Zara, shirt
Zara, skirt
Bex Rox, bracelet

Page 200
LK Bennett, dress
Topshop, denim jacket
J Crew, necklace
Made, bracelet

Wedding Belles
Page 219
Beulah, dress
Bionda Castana, heels
Mews London, necklace
Bag, stylists own
Accessorize, bag

The Art of Giving
Page 239
LK Bennett, top
Orelia, necklace

Grateful thanks to Denby
Pottery Company for the
tableware supplied on
pages 162, 166, 169, 171,
203, 207 and 213.

Also to Louise Taylor
Flowers for the
beautiful flowers seen
throughout this book.

Acknowledgements

First and foremost, thank you to my followers. Be it on YouTube, Instagram, Twitter or my blog, your support means the absolute world to me and none of this would be possible without your constant support and encouragement.

Thank you so much to all of the amazing people who helped bring this book to life... My management team at James Grant, Sophie Gildersleeve, Amy Newman (I miss you!) and Rory Scarfe, for working so hard to make this happen and making every meeting an absolute pleasure. To all of the wonderful team at Headline, especially my editor Rachel Kenny for staying so enthusiastic throughout and being an absolute pleasure to work with. A special thank you to Siobhan Hooper for once again bringing my vision to life and putting up with constant, extensive revisions and commentary on the design and styling of the book – you're a superstar!

To my good friend and hair magician Gareth Smith, incredibly kind and understanding stylist Emily Giffard-Taylor and once again to the fabulous Laurie Fletcher for making the photo shoots for this book so much fun!

Last but not least, thank you to my wonderful friends and family for supporting me always and keeping my feet firmly on the ground. You are everything to me. Mike, thank you for being the most understanding and kind person I've ever met. I adore you.

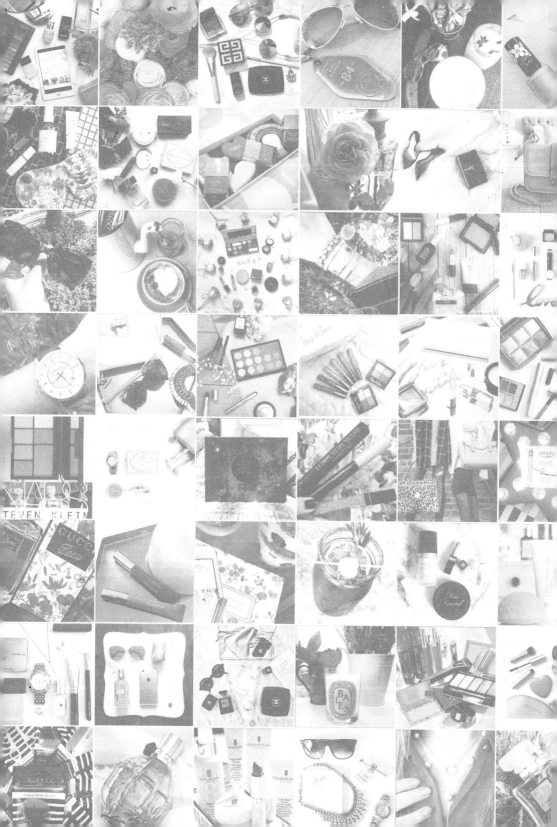